INTERMITTENT FASTING FOR WOMEN

A COMPLETE GUIDE TO FASTING FOR WEIGHT LOSS, BURN FAT AND IMPROVE THE QUALITY OF YOUR LIFE

ANTI-INFLAMMATORY DIET

THE ULTIMATE GUIDE TO HEAL THE IMMUNE SYSTEM, REDUCE INFLAMMATION AND WEIGHT LOSS WITH EASY AND HEALTHY RECIPES

2 books in 1: A Complete Guide to Weight Loss, Reduce Inflammation and Heal the Immune System

by Susan Lombardi

1

INTERMITTENT FASTING FOR WOMEN

A COMPLETE GUIDE TO FASTING FOR WEIGHT LOSS, BURN FAT AND IMPROVE THE QUALITY OF YOUR LIFE

By Susan Lombardi

Table of Contents

Introduction

Welcome to intermittent fasting for women! Thank you for finding this book worth your time and attention. Herein you'll find comprehensive information on intermittent fasting for women. The book elaborates how this form of fasting can transform your life by ushering you into a healthier lifestyle.

Whether you're hearing about intermittent fasting for the first time or have some information and you want to dig deeper, you will find chapter after chapter of comprehensive guidelines directing you on how to get into the fast and what to expect along the way.

This may be the first step on a long journey, to finally gaining the health, energy, vitality and gorgeous body that you've always dreamed of. The beauty of intermittent fasting is that it's very easy to use and works for most people. There are some folks that probably shouldn't use intermittent fasting and we'll discuss the issues with that in the book. But for most people, intermittent fasting is a great way to lose weight and feel great – as well as look your best.

Intermittent fasting will help you lose weight very rapidly and get your body into much better health than it is now. One of the problems that we have with the standard American diet is that too many people have insulin problems. You may not be diabetic, but you're probably suffering from problems related to insulin and blood sugar just the same.

Intermittent fasting can correct these problems very quickly. As you probably know, high insulin levels and more likely in overweight people.

More overweight you are, greater the amount of fat in your body and so your blood sugar levels also increases.

One of the goals of intermittent fasting is to jumpstart the metabolic system. Or maybe we should say it will reset the metabolic system, curing you of problems like insulin resistance. No matter what style of eating you choose, intermittent fasting can be very beneficial. Even better, intermittent fasting can correct these problems very quickly.

One of the reasons that intermittent fasting is becoming so popular is that it is very flexible. When you hear about fasting, you're probably thinking that it's some kind of hard-core idea that involves going days without eating. But this is it true at all. In fact, many types of intermittent fasting allow you to eat every single day. Some types of intermittent fasting, including the most popular ones, allow you to eat over a large time window during the day which means you can enjoy three square meals and even snacks. So you're hardly going to even notice that you're even fasting at all.

Another benefit of intermittent fasting is that it works with any kind of diet. Just go on YouTube and look for yourself. If you do, you'll see that many people get huge benefits from intermittent fasting without following any kind of diet. Some people are even eating junk food and losing huge amounts of weight. You'll see people eat all kinds of sugar and desserts, but if they do it over a very short time it doesn't affect their body weight or fat composition.

We only mention this to note that it's extremely flexible to use intermittent fasting. So you can go on eating the foods you're eating now, or if you want to maximize your weight loss, you can adopt a low-carb diet. But just keep in mind: you don't need to use a keto diet or any specific to enjoy the benefits of intermittent fasting.

Transformation is the most important word in this book. We will aim to keep transformation as the key goal – not only the transformation of our diet or health but a transformation of our entire lives. If this seems too far out of reach, do not be discouraged – it is easier than you think. Transformation does not require us to change who we truly are. We can keep all the things we love, but it will require a rewiring of how we view ourselves and the world around us. What could normally trigger a negative or detrimental attitude will be altered and viewed from a different perspective, a perspective that comes from a place of self-love and confidence. By applying the knowledge and practices we are about to learn into our lives, we can develop a lifestyle that will become second nature and only help us stay healthful physically and mentally.

In the chapters to come, we will discuss the ins and outs of Intermittent Fasting with an emphasis on women's weight loss in today's busy and complicated world. Women have to battle more difficulties than men for all of written history, and today there's no difference. Naturally, the extra stress on women to look and behave a certain way makes it very difficult to maintain balance during the mundane day-to-day tasks, thus making healthful lifestyles a choice that is overlooked or flat out cannot be obtained.

Chapter 1: What is Intermittent Fasting?

Intermittent Fasting is essentially the practice of restricting mealtimes, reducing snacking, or cutting out days of eating, based on the method one chooses. So many of us snack unconsciously or when we're getting moody without any real hunger. So many of us eat unconsciously in general, and then we're confused why our bodies are holding onto the weight. Intermittent Fasting reminds the body what food is for, and it restarts that nutritional absorption potential. All you have to do is cut out the snacks, fast a few hours a day, or just drink water a few days a week.

Intermittent Fasting (IF) is both a dietary choice and a lifestyle, but those who have the most success with IF will tell you that it became a lifestyle for them almost instantly. Sure, dieting plans and IF can match up nicely, but for some, IF requires no dietary change whatsoever. The point is to eat less and to eat less often. The brain and the body will respond in no time.

Practicing intermittent fasting helps strengthen our bodies to burn fat in contrast with our more common *fed* state. The body during the fed state relies on frequent resupplies of glucose and sugar for fuel. In addition to weight loss, stimulating and strengthening the metabolism provides numerous other health benefits that include enhanced mental clarity, focus, and stress reduction. The process and practice of intermittent fasting sharpens the mind and neural functions while reshaping the physical structure of our bodies at the cellular and molecular levels.

Whatever timeframe is chosen, the practice of intermittent fasting is possible to incorporate into daily life because it involves *fasting that occurs at irregular intervals* that are set by the individual and designed according to her preference.

This is the revolutionary secret of intermittent fasting: it can be tailored to the individual woman, rather than requiring her to conform to an extreme or unrealistic regime. This makes it fun and adaptable! You set the rules according to a plan that works for you.

Fasting is a relatively simple practice that yields incredible and complicated results. The effects that fasting has on the body and mind seems unfathomable: weight loss, blood sugar regulation, blood pressure regulation, and growth hormone regulation – only to name a few important ones. In recent years, science has reached full strength to support these claims, not to mention the thousands of online videos of people's results now that fasting has hit the mainstream. There are different types of fasting as well as many ways to fast.

Within the abundant array of different methods and individual changes any one person may implement, there is a wealth of potential ways to impact the health of the body and mind in positive ways. Fasting, in a general and broad definition, is the practice of willingly abstaining from something, usually food and drink. Whether it is simply not eating chocolate for a week or two or even cutting out all solid foods for a month, no matter how large or small the impact the abstinence has on you, that is fasting from your chosen food. Another more intensive fast would be dry fasting. Dry fasting is the complete abstinence from every source of solid or liquid food for any predetermined period, and, of course, willingly. Although not completely out of the question for beginners, these styles of fasting are used more sparingly than the style we aim to focus on, and that practice is called *Intermittent Fasting* or *IF* for short.

Chapter 2: Benefits of Intermittent Fasting

The main benefit of intermittent fasting is weight loss. However, there are several benefits of intermittent fasting, and most of them were widely recognized even in history.

In ancient times, fasting periods and seasons were referred to as cleanses, purifications or detoxifications, but the idea of all of them is the same. That is to do without eating food for a specified period. Ancient people believed that this period of fasting would clear their body systems of any toxin and rejuvenate them.

- Some of the most known benefits of intermittent fasting are:

Improved Mental Concentration and Clarity

Fasting has incredible benefits for the healthy function of the brain. The most known benefit stems from the activation of autophagy, which is a cell cleansing process. Note that fasting has anti-seizure effects.

Since the time immemorial human beings have been known to respond to caloric deprivation with a reduced size of major organs with two exemptions, the male testicles, and the brain.

This preservation of testicle size is a significant benefit because it helps to pass on genes to the next generation. Also, the of cognitive functions is essential for the survival of any human being.

For instance, imagine you are a caveman where food is scarce. When your brain starts to slow down the mental fog will make it harder to get food. Your brain power, one of the major advantages you have in the natural world, could be decreasing. Surviving without food will slowly erode your mental functioning until you are no longer able to perform essential blundering functions, let alone going out to get or to hunt food.

Therefore, for survival, cognitive functions in your body are maintained and boosted during fasting or starvation. This aspect has been known throughout the evolution of humankind. For instance, in ancient Greece, thinkers or scientists used to fast for days.

They fasted not because they wanted to lose some weight. They believed fasting would increase and improve their mental agility. Even today, people marvel at the ancient Greek mathematicians and philosophers. Even in the history of Japanese prisoners during the Second World War people have been describing the unquestionable clarity of thought that accompanies starvation and fasting. This book describes a prisoner who would read several books from his memory and another prisoner who mastered the Norwegian language in a few days.

Healthier Way to Lose Weight

Intermittent fasting is a healthier way for people to lose weight. As a result of the flexibility of this diet, you are still able to continue consuming everything that is healthy for you. Any dietary considerations that you may need to accommodate for can easily be taken into consideration and accounted for with intermittent fasting. This makes it easy and effortless when it comes to losing weight.

Unlike other diets, there are no restricting calories or starving yourself with the intermittent fasting diet. You will not experience any sensations of hunger or feeling as though you are not getting enough. Whereas other diets are often not able to be maintained for long, resulting in unhealthy practices of yo-yo dieting, intermittent fasting can be. This means that the diet is not only healthier but also more sustainable.

When you are eating the intermittent fasting diet, you can look forward to losing fat specifically. This diet supports you in letting go of unwanted tummy fat and other fat on your body that may be stubborn and resistant to other diets. Intermittent fasting is both healthier and more effective in supporting you with reaching your weight loss goals.

Supports Healthy Bodily Functions

Intermittent fasting gives your body time to complete processes and functions before introducing more food into your system. This means that every time you eat, you are giving your body adequate time to actually metabolize the food and use it appropriately. In modern society, we regularly overeat and push our bodies to constantly be in a state of digesting. As a result, our systems become overwhelmed and we do not effectively metabolize everything. This can lead to you not getting enough nutrition, storing fats, and struggling to produce healthy levels of natural hormones and chemicals within your body.

When you eat the intermittent fasting diet, you support your body by giving it enough time to process everything. As a result, its ability to metabolize food and gain everything from it is improved. Your insulin levels drop significantly, which supports your body in burning fat. You also notice an increase in human growth hormone that can reach up to 5x your original value. This supports you in fat burning as well as muscle gain. As a result of your intermittent fasting, your body is able to focus more energy on other processes beyond digesting food. This means that things like cellular repair functions have a greater ability to take place. So, your body has a stronger ability in removing waste materials from your cells and supporting them in healing from any damage that they may experience. Finally, intermittent fasting is known for supporting people with gene expression. This means that this dietary habit can support your genes in changing in ways that actually protect them against diseases and promote a longer lifespan. Your body has a much stronger ability to remain healthy and function optimally when you eat according to the intermittent fasting diet.

Supports You in Healing Faster

When your cells have an easier time restoring themselves and your body is exposed to less stress, you have an easier time in healing faster. This means that any time you place a physical strain on your body, you can look forward to spending less time healing from that experience.

This is beneficial for many reasons. One of the biggest reasons, however, is that when you are able to heal faster you are able to increase your health faster. Activities such as working out and lifting weights require your body to take some downtime to heal in between. Any time you are seeking to increase your muscular strength, you will experience ripping in your muscles. Then, the muscle tissue heals and grows back in a greater quantity. This is what leads to muscle growth. It is also what leads to pain after working out.

When you eat according to the intermittent fasting diet, your ability to heal from this type of damage is improved. This means that you can gain muscle faster and without having a negative impact on your overall health.

In addition to intentional healing that is required after activities such as working out, you will also have an easier time healing from other physical ailments. For example, if you endure an accidental injury your body will have an easier time healing it than it would if you were in ill health. Because your body has an improved ability to repair cells, you can look forward to healing much quicker from any injury that you might experience.

You Can Maintain a More Youthful Appearance

Improved cellular repairs and gene expression is not only great for healing, but it is also great for maintaining a youthful vitality! When these functions improve for you, your body's ability to maintain healthier skin, hair, nails, and other bodily features is improved, too. This means that you can look forward to maintaining a more youthful appearance just by adjusting your diet and eating the intermittent fasting way.

In addition to actually looking more youthful, you can also enjoy the experience of feeling more youthful, too. People who eat the intermittent fasting diet report feeling greater levels of energy. As a result, they are able to start enjoying life with a greater vitality about them. This means that you can enjoy all of the activities that you have been missing as a result of low energy and ill health, like dancing and spending time enjoying life with your loved ones!

Lowers Your Risk of Contracting Diseases

When your immune system is operating optimally and your entire bodily functions are improved, you can enjoy the benefits of lowered risk of contracting diseases. As you already know, diseases like type 2 diabetes, Alzheimer's, and cancer have been prevented by the intermittent fasting diet. However, this diet can also support you in preventing other potential diseases, too.

Eating the intermittent fasting diet has proven to level out blood pressure, reduce bad cholesterol, lower inflammatory markers, and lower blood sugar levels in your blood. This means that you can look forward to having better heart health. You also work toward preventing heart disease by eating this way.

Reduced instances of inflammation markers also mean that the intermittent fasting diet can also support you in preventing or curing symptoms of diseases like fibromyalgia. They can also support you in healing from chronic fatigue syndrome, and other conditions that are typically related to poor inner health.

Your improved diet will also support your healthy brain functions. When you eat in accordance with the intermittent fasting diet, you also support the growth of new nerve cells, as well as a brain-derived neurotrophic factor (BDNF.) Both of these instances can support you in improving brain health and function overall. This means that you are at a lower risk of experiencing clinical depression, or that you may even be able to reverse the symptoms that you have already experienced. Furthermore, this can also support you in recovering from any damage that could be experienced as a result of a stroke.

Reduces Inflammation and Physical Stress

The intermittent fasting diet is known to eliminate free radicals from your body. This means that you are less likely to experience chronic inflammation and physical stress that is based on nutrition and nourishment.

For many people, chronic inflammation and physical stress that is derived from nourishment can be the root cause of many physical symptoms. Often, people go undiagnosed yet continue to experience frustrating symptoms like pain, swelling, headaches, and metabolic issues when they experience chronic inflammation. This can be frustrating and can lead to a feeling of hopelessness and anger when it comes to trying to resume a healthy and active lifestyle. Intermittent fasting may be able to support you in overcoming these symptoms if they are being caused by chronic inflammation or physical stress.

May Extend Your Lifespan

Intermittent fasting has shown in some studies that it may be able to extend your lifespan. Many people find themselves living shorter lives with poorer quality of life as a result of poor health. Disease and illness kill far more people each year than actual old age or natural causes do. Using the intermittent fasting diet may support you in preventing these illnesses and diseases so that you can live a longer, healthier, natural life.

Although this has not yet been tested in humans, the intermittent fasting diet was tested in lab rats. Through these tests, some studies showed that the rats lived as much as 83% longer than those who did not fast. Despite this specific piece of evidence not yet being tested on humans, there is plenty of evidence that suggests that the factors that prevent longer and healthier lives can be avoided with intermittent fasting. For this reason, we can assume that intermittent fasting may indeed support humans in living longer and healthier lives, too.

Boosts Your Immune System

As a result of the many benefits that you gain from intermittent fasting, you also get to look forward to having an improved immune system. This is from the combination of reduced physical stress, increased cellular reparation abilities, weight loss, and other benefits that you gain from intermittent fasting.

Your boosted immune system will be supportive in preventing you from experiencing long-term health conditions such as various illnesses and diseases. It will also support you in preventing the contraction of less dangerous illnesses such as the common cold and influenza. As a result, you can look forward to spending less time being sick and more time on your feet and enjoying life.

Increased Ketones

Fasting for anywhere from 10-16 hours every single day is said to improve your body's ability to release ketones into your bloodstream. This releasing of ketones encourages your body to consume and burn fat rather than carbohydrates when it comes to producing energy for you throughout the day. This means that using the intermittent fasting diet supports weight loss through actually using your fatty weight as a fuel.

Many people actually choose to combine intermittent fasting with the keto diet as a way to increase weight loss. Furthermore, they find that these two combined eating styles result in them feeling greater energy levels, having healthier bodily functions, and experiencing greater mental clarity. There are many benefits that can be gained from intermittent fasting alone, but when you combine it with the keto diet it can truly be life-changing!

Mental Sharpness and Intermittent Fasting

Consider and think about the large Thanksgiving turkey and pumpkin pie. After that meal, were you mentally sharp? Or were you dull? What about the opposite when you were hungry? Were you slothful and tired? The answer is a big no. When you were hungry, your senses were hyper-alert, and your mind was very sharp. The fact that consuming food would make you concentrate even better is not true. There are survival advantages to human beings that are cognitively sharp. You will also experience physical agility when you are fasting.

When you say that you are hungry for something, such as hungry for attention, hungry for power, does it mean that you are dull and slothful? It does not mean that. It means that your mind is energetic and hyper-vigilant. Hunger and fasting activate you toward your goal. Many people tend to think that fasting would dull their senses, but the truth is that it has an energizing effect.

Therefore, there will be an increase in your brain connectivity and some new neuron growth in your stem cells. This is mediated in part by your brain-derived neurotrophic factor. For women, both fasting and exercise increase brain-derived neurotrophic factor expression in many parts of their brain. BDNF plays a major role in glucose metabolism, appetite, and control of gastrointestinal and cardiovascular systems.

Intermittent Fasting & Neurodegenerative Disorders

There is also another aspect of neurodegenerative diseases and fasting. If you maintain intermittent fasting, you will experience less age-related deterioration of neurons as compared to a person who is on a normal diet. You will also experience fewer symptoms in diseases such as Huntington's, Parkinson's, and Alzheimer's disease.

The benefits of intermittent fasting to your brain can be experienced in both during caloric restriction and fasting. During calorie restriction and exercise, you will experience increased electrical and synaptic activity in your brain.

Intermittent Fasting and Alzheimer's Disorders

These complications are characterized by an abnormal accumulation of proteins in the body cells. There are two classes of Alzheimer's disorders, neurofibrillary tangles and amyloid plaques. The known symptoms of Alzheimer's disorders closely correlate with the accumulation of these tangles and plagues. These abnormal protein accumulations in the body cells are believed to negatively affect the synaptic connections in your memory and the cognition parts of your brain.

Some specific proteins such as HSP-70 are known to prevent damages and misfolding of amyloid and neurofibrillary tangles proteins. Therefore alternate fasting will increase the levels of HSP-70 protein. When amyloid and tau proteins are destroyed beyond repair, they are removed by autophagy. This process is accelerated by Intermittent Fasting.

Intermittent Fasting and Breast Cancer

Low-calorie meals are a strategy to prevent breast cancer. It has beneficial effects on the overall health of breast cells within the breasts of a woman. Overweight women have large fat cells in their breasts, and this increases the amount of estrogen within the breast. They can also store fats in their liver and in their abdomen where it increases the circulation of sex hormones, insulin hormone, inflammation and fat produced hormones. These changes leads to the development of breast cancer.

Intermittent Fasting and Insulin Sensitivity

As far as metabolism of glucose is concerned, intermittent fasting is perfect. It is a powerful tool that normalizes glucose. It also improves the glucose variability.

Chapter 3: Intermittent Fasting Techniques

Now that we have discussed how your body will react to fasting let's discuss the many different forms of fasting. Although there are seemingly infinite ways to go about your Intermittent Fasting routine, we will focus on six methods that are popular among fitness experts and the fasting community. We will discuss the suitable timing of 'eating windows', the duration of time in the day when you are allowed to eat, and compare each method so you can successfully choose the best one for your lifestyle. Although fasting has its roots in religion and spirituality, we will not go extensively into these practices, but if you wish to combine your spiritual goals with these methods, you can go right ahead.

At this point, we would like to state that keeping a fasting notebook helps immensely for someone just starting out. By recording our experiences and documenting how successful or unsuccessful our routine is, we can find insight into ourselves and also organize the aspects of our routine that may need to be altered or customized. It is not mandatory to have a notebook, but throughout this book, we will be keeping track of our experiences and analyzing our regimen to understand better what works for us as individuals.

The 16/8 Method

Also known as the *Leangain's method*, this method was popularized by Martin Berkhan. The eating window for this style is eight hours with a sixteen-hour fasting time. So if you sleep eight hours, awake, then restrict caloric intake for eight hours, then you can eat as much as you like until bedtime. Another example would be to awake, start your eight-hour eating window, then begin fasting for the evening and during sleep. This is a common choice for people who already skip breakfast. Tea and coffee have no calories, so they are still allowed to be consumed, obviously without sugar added.

Overview:

- *Sixteen hours of fasting*

- *Eight-hour consumption window*

- *Zero-calorie drinks allowed*

The 5/2 Diet Method

This method looks more like a diet than a proper fast, but it is a popular method for weight loss and often finds its way into IF circles. First popularized by Michael Mosley, it is also called the 'Fast Diet'. This method involves your normal eating routine for five days of the week then restricting your caloric intake to 600 calories or less for two days of the week. So you can choose your two days to fast whether they are together or not, let's say Wednesday and Friday. Then, treat all other days as normal days, but on Wednesday and Friday, you eat one or two small meals that together equal 600 calories or less. This is a great beginner diet to try before you get into some more intensive IF. If you're wary of how you may react to fasting, then this method is great to start.

- *Five days of normal meals according to your daily diet*

- *Two days of consuming 600 calories or less*

The Eat Stop Eat Method

That is 24 hours of no solid food or caloric intake. Unsweetened coffee and tea are acceptable during the fasting days for this method. A great example would be to fast from dinner to dinner or, let's say, from 4:00 pm to 4:00 pm the next day. It does not matter what time frame you choose, but it should be a solid 24-hour period. Keeping to your usual eating schedule on the non-fasting days is important.

Overview:

- *Strict 24-hour fast once or twice a week*

- *Maintain usual eating schedule during non-fast days*

Lean-Gains Method (14:10)

The lean-gains method has several different incarnations on the web, but its fame comes from the fact that it helps shed fat while building it into muscle almost immediately. Through the lean-gains method, you'll find yourself able to shift all that fat to be muscle through a rigorous practice of fasting, eating right, and exercising.

Through this method, you fast anywhere from 14 to 16 hours and then spend the remaining 10 or 8 hours each day engaged in eating and exercise. This method, as opposed to the crescendo, features daily fasting and eating, rather than alternated days of eating versus not. Therefore, you don't have to be quite so cautious about extending the physical effort to exercise on the days you are fasting because those days when you're fasting are literally every day!

For the lean-gains method, start fasting only 14 hours and work it up to 16 if you feel comfortable with it, but never forget to drink enough water and be careful about expending too much energy on exercise! Remember that you want to grow in health and potential through intermittent fasting. You'll certainly not want to lose any of that growth by forcing the process along.

Crescendo Method

This is usually an introduction to fasting, it is how many people begin their fasting journey. This is a less intense form of intermittent fasting and is a great way for you to see how it works to ease your fears and become familiarized with a fasting schedule. This method involves normally for 4 or 5 days a week and then restricting your eating period to between 8 or 10 hours for two or three non-consecutive days. Very similar to the 16/8 method, but instead of doing every day, you only do it a couple days each week. These are the safest ways for women to fast because they do not upset the hormonal balance of the body. Intermittent fasting not done properly can trick the body into going into what is known as starvation mode. This happens when the body thinks it needs to hold onto fat longer because it doesn't know when it will have a chance to consume food for fuel again. This can lead to burning muscle for fuel as well as upsetting the hormonal balance, leading to even more issues. However, intermittent fasting done properly can be safe and incredibly beneficial.

Not only does intermittent fasting help you lose weight, but it also improves mental clarity and allows you to simplify your life in a way that diets do not. Think about how much time you spend worrying about or eating food, and then imagine what other things you could be doing if this were not the case. This is one the major benefits of intermittent fasting, there are no surprises and you are able to take complete control of when you eat.

The Alternating Day Method

This method involves fasting every other day. This method can be customized to your liking on the fast days. You can cut back to 600 calories a day, not unlike the 5/2 method, but fasting every other day. If you feel comfortable, you can intake zero calories on the fast days; this would be a very intense method and is not recommended for beginners. For example, eat normally on Sunday, lower calorie intake to 600 calories or less on Monday, eat normally on Tuesday, lower calorie intake Wednesday, eat normally on Thursday, lower calories on Friday. You see, we hit a snag in our pattern as there is an odd number of days in a week. For the odd day out, in this case, Saturday, you can choose to lower the calorie count or eat regularly. It is up to you. For another example, the Saturday odd day out, you could potentially fast for 24 hours then jump back into the pattern on Sunday.

Overview:

- *Fast or lower calories every other day*

- *Keep a usual eating schedule on non-fast days*

- *Choose what suits you best for the odd day out*

The Warrior Method

This method was popularized by Ori Hofmekler. It includes eating small amounts of raw plant-based foods during the day, then one large meal during the evening. Essentially, you are fasting all day and breaking the fast at night. This diet typically focuses on eating raw and unprocessed foods to get the full benefit. For example, during the day, you snack on fruits, veggies, and nuts. Once the evening comes, you prepare a large meal that is as unprocessed and raw as possible.

Overview:

- *Light amounts of raw foods or completely fasting during daylight hours*

- *A large meal at night, as unprocessed and raw as possible*

20:4 Method

Stepping things up a notch from the 14:10 and 16:8 methods, the 20:4 method is a tough one to master, for it is rather unforgiving. People talk about this method of intermittent fasting as intense and highly restrictive, but they also say that the effects of living this method are almost unparalleled with all other tactics.

For the 20:4 method, you'll fast for 20 hours each day and squeeze all your meals, all your eating, and all your snacking into 4 hours. People who attempt 20:4 normally have two smaller meals or just one large meal and a few snacks during their 4-hour window to eat, and it really is up to the individual which four hours of the day they devote to eating.

The trick for this method is to make sure you're not overeating or bingeing during those 4-hour windows to eat. It is all-too-easy to get hungry during the 20-hour fast and have that feeling then propel you into intense and unrealistic hunger or meal sizes after the fast period is over. Be careful if you try this method. If you're new to intermittent fasting, work your way up to this one gradually, and if you're working your way up already, only make the shift to 20:4 when you know you're ready. It would surely disappoint if all your progress with intermittent fasting got hijacked by one poorly thought-out goal with 20:4 method.

Meal Skipping

Meal skipping is an extremely flexible form of intermittent fasting that can provide all of the benefits of intermittent fasting but with less of the strict scheduling. If you are not someone who has a typical schedule or who feels as though a more strict variation of the intermittent fasting diet will serve you, meal skipping is a viable alternative.

Many people who choose to use meal skipping find it to be a great way to listen to their body and follow their basic instincts. If they are not hungry, they simply don't eat that meal. Instead, they wait for the next one. Meal skipping can also be helpful for people who have time constraints and who may not always be able to get in a certain meal of the day.

It is important to realize that with meal skipping, you may not always be maintaining a 10-16-hour window of fasting. As a result, you may not get every benefit that comes from other fasting diets. However, this may be a great solution to people who want an intermittent fasting diet that feels more natural to them. It may also be a great idea for those who are looking to begin listening to their body more so that they can adjust to a more intense variation of the diet with greater ease. In other words, it can be a great transitional diet for you if you are not ready to jump into one of the other fasting diets just yet.

The Spontaneity Method

This method is the loosest and most flexible method of IF. The method is pretty straight forward; there are no guidelines or structures. Simply skip a meal when it's convenient or if you're not hungry. Skipping one or two meals every so often can be a great foundation to lay while you search for a more suitable routine. This method also comes in handy for busy people, parents, or just people who love winging it.

Overview:

- *No structure*

- *Simply skip meals when convenient, or fast whenever you like*

Now that we have a general idea of different fasting techniques, keep in mind that these are guidelines that can be customized to fit your specific lifestyle. To reiterate: no one way suits everyone. So as you analyze these methods, keep in mind your personal life and how you alter the structures not only to fit into your schedule but also to personalize your practice. By personalizing your routine, you allow yourself some added empowerment and something that you helped create. Some examples of customizing your practice can include changing the length of fasts, changing diet to suit (vegan, Paleo, etc.), and/or changing the fasting patterns (alternating every two days, etc.). With the methods above, we see many similarities between them. With the main premise being a caloric restriction and eating window restriction, these methods are simply different customized versions of fasting itself. So this means that we can customize these methods to suit our needs and preferences as individuals.

When we decide to customize a method, it needs to be well thought out. *Why do I need these customizations? Are these customizations feasible as something I can accomplish?* There is an infinite number of ways we can change and alter these techniques, and we will provide some examples below. Keep in mind these are not the only ways to customize but just some basic strategies.

Customize as you please, but be safe and mindful in doing so:

- **Customization Strategy #1**: *Altering the duration of eating windows*

We see above that one of the main differences in these methods is the timing. For example, the 16/8 method requires eating for eight hours of the day and fasting for sixteen hours of the day. This can be altered easily to suit you. Need a little extra time for the eating window? Add an hour. Feeling confident that you can shorten the eating window? Shorten it an hour or two. You can also choose your eating window during the day. Morning, midday or night are all suitable times to eat depending on your schedule.

- **Customization Strategy #2**: *Altering days*

Days in which you choose to fast are very important but not limited to the guidelines above. The alternating method as an example, alternating days of fasting is a simple pattern, but what if you need two days off from fasting? Make your fast days every third day. Another example would be putting more fast days together, as with the Eat Stop Eat method. Instead of one or two days of complete calorie restriction, maybe do three or push your two days back-to-back for a more challenging fast.

- ***Customization Strategy #3***: *Altering the timing of meals*

Much content online will suggest a proper time for having your meals or will cite the warrior method as an example that requires a large meal at night. This large meal can be placed anywhere in the day according to your preference; in fact, many people prefer their large meal in the middle of the day to avoid a full stomach while sleeping.

- **Customization strategy #4**: *Altering meal choices*

As noted above, the warrior method requires raw foods to be ingested. Many people have dietary restrictions and preferences that may not fit into these diets and methods, so switch it up! What you eat during your IF routines is important, and you want to keep it healthy. But be reasonable with yourself; choose foods you enjoy. If you prefer fried, greasy foods, maybe try the same ingredients but prepared differently – baked chicken instead of breaded and fried, *etc.*

- **Customization strategy #5**: *Include your lifestyle*

When we research fasting online, we see a pattern – health blogs with muscular people in their fitness attire smiling brightly in front of a sunset. This is all fine for some people, but many do not relate to this lifestyle. Lucky for us, fasting is for everyone. You can add fasting to your normal routine easily without hitting the gym or buying spandex. Make it a point to meld IF into your lifestyle rather than view it as something separate from you. Any hobby you love – gaming, fishing, reading, music, art, scrapbooking, *etc.* – can be a part of your fasting routine. In fact, having a low-intensity hobby is great for the downtime during fasts.

Chapter 4: Choosing the right fasting regime

When you make your choice from the different options listed above, there are several things you'll want to keep in mind. First and foremost, amongst those things will be the fact that you can always choose another method (or a more flexible one to start with) in case something doesn't work as you'd hoped.

Ultimately, you'll also want to keep the following points in mind as you go about selecting your method: body type & abilities, lifestyle, daily tendencies, work routine, friends & family, and dietary choices. For all these considerations, remember what feels best to you, and remember to keep your goals with IF in mind at all times!

Consider your body type and abilities:
Think of how your body looks and feels and how much about it you'd like to change. Think about how you react to food and what it looks like when you're hungry. Think about those things you view as your "limits" and how comfortable you are with pushing. Are you a fitness freak or a couch potato? Are you huskier or slimmer? Does your body hold onto fat or build muscle quickly? Do you retain water weight or not? Do you work out? Do you require a lot of water when you do? Consider all these things about your body and more, then compare them to the methods listed above.

Consider your lifestyle:

When do you normally wake up and how much sleep do you get on an average night? How hungry are you normally when you do wake up? How fast is your metabolism and when do you notice its peak? How do you make your living? Do you spend a lot of time in the car or on your feet or in an office? Are you constantly around other people or are you often alone? When you choose your method for Intermittent Fasting, make sure to consider all these lifestyle points. Maybe you wouldn't want to choose a method that forces you to eat when you're supposed to be at work.

Consider your daily tendencies:

Do you eat mostly in the daylight hours or after the sun goes down? Do you go to work in the daytime or night time? Are you generally nocturnal, diurnal, or crepuscular? Do you have a lot of freedom and flexibility in your daily routines? Do you travel a lot for work? Do you spend a lot of time on the move? Do you have trouble remembering to eat? Are you the type of person that works out on the regular? Consider these themes in your life and more before you choose your method. Does it make sense for you to have low intake days where you consume 500 calories or less? Or does it make more sense for you to have extended periods in each day where you're just not eating based on your habits or tendencies or otherwise? Plan something that makes sense and respects your habits so that the transition into Intermittent Fasting is as easy and painless as possible.

Consider your work routine:

Do you go to work in the morning or night? Are you allowed to eat at work? Do you work around food or in the food service industry? Do you work on your feet all day or by doing something strenuous? Do you receive purposeful or accidental exercise opportunities at work or are you just sitting in the same position all day? All these elements of your work routine will be important to consider as you decide which avenue of Intermittent Fasting to go down. You won't want to engage in a method like 20:4 if you're at work every day for incredibly short shifts. 20:4 works better for someone who works very long and distracting days. You won't want to try a method like 12:12 if part of your eating window involves being at work, when you're not allowed to eat at work. Remember to take your work life, routines, and restrictions into account when you go about making this choice, for you will make things much less harsh on yourself if you can look at this bigger picture from the beginning and planning stages.

Consider your friends, co-workers, and family:

How loud are their opinions? Are their lives oriented toward health? Do they demean you a lot or make fun of your choices? Or are they encouraging all the time? Are these people your support system or are they your devils' advocates? Do you have the sense that they want to see you succeed? On the most basic level, are they nice to you and respectful of your choices? It might not seem that important, but the attitudes and supportive capacity of your friends, co-workers, and family can mean the world when you make a big choice like starting Intermittent Fasting in your life. Sometimes, people just don't want to see us succeed. They block our successes with jealousy, pride, ignorance, or arrogance. When friends and family act like this, it's better to choose a method that allows you to avoid discussing IF around them whatsoever. When friends and family are open and supportive, they shouldn't influence your choice that much at all; it's just when things are tenuous that you'll need to keep them (and your time around them) in consideration.

Consider your dietary choices:

Do you eat a lot of processed foods? Or do you eat a largely whole-foods, plant-based diet? Do you count calories? Do you cautiously skim nutrition facts? Are you looking for something specific like high fat, high fiber, or high protein? Are you hoping to change your diet entirely or are you trying to keep things the way they are? Are you willing to sacrifice items of your diet to actualize your goals?

All these questions help determine which type of method you're going to be ready for.

Essentially, if you're trying to change your diet entirely, a method with days "on" and days "off" will work best for you. In this case, try 5:2, alternate-day, eat-stop-eat, and spontaneous skip methods.

However, if you don't want to change your diet that much at all, a method where you fast for periods within each day will be desirable instead. Try methods like 20:4, 16:8, 14:10, or 12:12 for this type of situation.

As long as you make your selection with these points in mind, you're sure to succeed with your Intermittent Fasting goals. You enable yourself to make the safest, smartest, best choice for your circumstances, and that's an incredible tool to use in so many different applications. In this case, it's a tool that will help keep you healthy, boost your brain, heal your heart, and shed that excess weight like melted butter!

Chapter 5: Effects of Intermittent Fasting

There are <u>pros and cons</u> of everything and intermittent fasting is no exception. It's a complete lifestyle change and hence making the transition can be difficult for some people. This section will help you in understanding how intermittent fasting can impact your health positively and the problems that you can face and how to deal with them.

Positive Impacts

Detoxification:

Whether you lose weight, or not, and how much weight you lose, is irrelevant inasmuch as the detoxing effect that intermittent fasting has on the body. You see, we accumulate toxins in our bodies over time. We tend to pick them up from food, air, drinks, and basically anything we come into contact with. These toxins enter the body and the immune system hacks away at them.

Generally speaking, the immune system will beat up toxins and rid the body of these harmful substances. However, the immune system needs certain freedom in order to function at full speed. Since the immune system is part of the overall human body machinery, it needs energy just like the other systems in the body.

Therefore, it essentially competes for energy. And when other systems in the body are overloaded, the immune system tends to become overwhelmed.

So, when the fasting process begins, the digestive tract begins to clear excess matter, including build up, until the digestive tract becomes clear of residue. This is part of the detoxification process. The body is now clearing waste that it doesn't need.

This process of clearing excess matter gives the immune system a chance to catch and fight off toxins as there are no new toxins coming in for a specific amount of time.

As the body begins to detox, the waste expelled from the organism allows organ systems to function better, the blood is improved, kidneys and liver function also improves, while high blood pressure may begin to dissipate. If this can be followed up with a balanced diet on non-fast days, then you could be setting yourself up for a dramatic turnaround which can leave you feeling like a million bucks.

Weight Loss:

The biggest reason why people engage in the intermittent fasting movement is because they are looking to lose weight. Well, first, I'd like to point out that losing weight is not the underlying intent of people who begin with intermittent fasting. Their true intention is to look better and feel better about themselves. And that does not necessarily imply that you need to lose weight.

In fact, crash diets have a habit of forcing the body to burn muscle instead of fat. So, dieters feel that the crash diet is working but in reality, all they are doing is changing their body composition. They are substituting lean muscle for fat. Naturally, muscle weighs more than fat. And so, the "benefits" are seen by the dieter.

But these results are not actually healthy results. They are simply a change in body composition which, in the end, leads to the rebound effect among other dietary conditions.

However, the intermittent fasting approach calls for the body to use up excess stores. This function is also improved when the individual is able to detox. So, the digestive system works much more efficiently. In turn, this kicks the metabolism into high gear giving it a chance to catch up.

Improved Blood Sugar Levels:

Speaking of blood sugar levels, intermittent fasting has been linked to improving blood sugar levels. While the data on this claim is still a bit sketchy, it seems to support the fact that the lack of caloric intake, especially sugars, will enable to body to detox and begin to process intake a lot better as compared to regular eating days.

This implies that the body is able to regular blood sugar to normal levels thereby reducing the overload that high amounts of sugar may cause on the body. In turn, this allows insulin production to level off and revert many of the adverse effects of having high blood sugar.

This regulatory effect allows the body to begin recovering its natural functions thereby improving overall wellness. Truth be told, high blood sugar levels are a real killer since they make it very hard for the body to level out hormonal function especially when insulin is out of whack. So, intermittent fasting is definitely an alternative for those folks who have high blood sugar levels and are looking to improve their body's overall ability to process sugar.

Effect on High Blood Pressure:
Another interesting effect stemming from intermittent fasting is on high blood pressure.

In general, high blood pressure is associated with high levels of consumption in fat and sodium, that is, salt. When this happens, the body may trigger a reaction by elevating blood pressure in order to compensate for the constricted blood vessels.

Intermittent fasting, as has been stated, helps the body detox. And sodium (salt) is one of the most complex toxins in the body.

Sodium is soluble and water and is usually excreted in the urine. However, when sodium levels surpass the kidneys filtering capabilities, then one of the responses, in addition to water retention, is elevated blood pressure.

This condition will trigger the kidneys to work overtime in order to reduce the excess sodium in the body. This is where an individual may experience acute kidney failure, and if care is not taken, may lead to chronic kidney failure.

Effects on Heart Health:
Heart health is a complicated issue in today's world. We all want to be healthy and thrive, but the foods we eat and the activities we engage in often don't align with those goals, and those more immediate actions win out. In effect, many of our hearts aren't as healthy as they could be. Heart

disease is still the biggest killer in the world to this day. However, the introduction of Intermittent Fasting into someone's lifestyle can greatly alter this potential, for it can reduce many risks associated with heart disease.

When it comes down to it, as long as one's Intermittent Fasting experience involves the reintroduction of electrolytes into the body, there's no potential harm posed to the heart whatsoever. There's only potential for growth, bolstering, and strengthening. However, without the right reintroduction of electrolytes, there *is* still the possibility of heart palpitations in individuals attempting IF. The heart needs electrolytes for its stability and efficacy, so as long as you drink a bit of salt with your water, your heart will only thank you!

Intermittent Fasting and Aging:

People love to talk about how Intermittent Fasting can reverse the effects of aging, and they're not wrong! The tricky part is elucidating the science behind the process they're referencing. The anti-aging potential tied up with Intermittent Fasting applies mostly to two things, your brain and, your whole body, through what's called "*autophagy*". Overall, Intermittent Fasting heals the body through its ability to rejuvenate the cells. With this restricted caloric intake due to eating schedule or timing, the body's cells can function with less limitation and confusion while producing more energy for the body to use. In effect, the cells function more efficiently while the body can burn more fat and take in more oxygen for the organs and blood, encouraging the individual to live longer with increased sensations of "youth." Intermittent Fasting has been proven to keep the brain fit and agile. It improves overall cognitive function and memory capacity as well as cleverness, wit, and quick, clear thinking in the moment. Furthermore, Intermittent Fasting keeps the cells fit and agile through autophagy which is kick started by intermittent fasting where the cells are encouraged to clean themselves up and get rid of any "trash" that might be clogging up the works. By restricting your eating schedule a little bit each day (or each week), you can find your brain power boosted and your body ready for anything.

Side Effects

Headache:

It is the most common problem that people face. There is nothing to worry about the headaches as they occur when you are going through sugar withdrawal systems.

Our lifestyle has become such that our dependency on a carbohydrate-rich diet has increased a lot. We also keep consuming meals at frequent intervals and hence our body keeps getting glucose supply at short intervals. Our body loves glucose fuel as it is easy to burn and can be absorbed by the cells directly. However, being easy doesn't make it good. It leaves a lot of waste and residue in the body.

When you begin intermittent fasting, you block the regular supply of glucose fuel. Your body requires energy dump at short intervals. It can also derive energy from the fat stores but it is difficult to burn fuel and hence your brain starts giving you signals to eat frequently in the form of a headache. If you don't start eating frequently, your body would have no other option than to switch to fat fuel in the body. It is a clean fuel, leaves no toxic waste and residue. It would make you slimmer and also help in getting rid of diseases.

The easy way to counter the headaches is to have unsweetened black tea or coffee. These beverages help in dealing with the headache and also don't add any calorie to your system. You can have them without breaking your fast.

Hunger Pangs:

As we have already discussed in the book, the hunger pangs are a function of your biological clock. Even if you are feeling hungry it doesn't mean that you need to eat. The feeling of hunger is created by the release of a hormone called *Ghrelin*. The gut releases this hormone at times when you have food in a normal routine. It means that if you are habitual of eating at 8 in the morning or you eat immediately after brushing, you would feel the urge to eat at these times. The Ghrelin release is triggered by these signals. It wouldn't matter much that you had eaten a short while ago. The Ghrelin release is also triggered by time and incidents and not just by hunger. Now, because the hunger pangs are more dependent on signals than actual hunger they can be shifted easily. Another important thing about hunger pangs is that they are short. It means that if you are having hunger pangs, stomach cramps, and other such symptoms, you'll only need to hold on to it for a short while and they'll subside. Diverting your attention toward other important things is also a good way to avoid hunger pangs. Physical activities like walking, jogging and swimming can also help in subsiding hunger pangs. If you want, you can also drink unsweetened fresh lime water, black tea or coffee without sugar or water to fill your stomach and it would also help in suppressing the hunger. Very soon your gut will get used to the changed schedule and you will stop getting troubled by the hunger pangs.

Cravings:

Cravings can mean a lot of different things for men but they have a completely unique meaning when it comes to women. Food cravings can arise in women due to emotional needs or psychological distress too. Women can find great solace in food, especially in sweets and desserts.

However, craving, in general, is bad and the biggest cause of food craving is the intake of sweets. Candies, chocolates, cookies, carbonated beverages and other such things that are high in sugar content can cause sugar cravings. You must always try to stay away from such things.

There are <u>several reasons</u> because this happens:

- These things add lots of calories to your system and it can be counterproductive when you are trying to lose weight

- Most sweets have very high sugar content and low fiber. Although these things would give a signal to your system that a lot of calories are coming, your gut would get nothing in reality. However, the release of digestive juices would be there. It would harm your system seriously.

- The more sweets you eat, the faster you'll feel the need to eat again. Refined sugar is more addictive than most addictive substances in this world.

- High sugar foods would make you feel fuller very fast but they would also make you feel empty stomach with the same speed. This is highly confusing for your gut and your blood sugar control system also remains engaged unnecessarily.

The best way to deal with these problems is to abstain from high sugar foods completely. If possible staying away from high carb food items is also highly advisable as they also have a lot of sugar. You must try to avoid processed food items as much as possible.

Eat food items that are high in healthy fats and proteins. The higher the fat and protein content in your food, the lower will be your food cravings and these nutrients take a lot of time to get processed in the gut. Your gut remains pleasantly engaged and is able to clean itself properly.

Frequent Trips to the Toilet:

It is not very unusual for people to feel the frequent need to urinate when they begin their fasting routine. However, there is no need to worry as it is common for most weight loss programs. When you start any weight loss program and reduce your calorie intake, your body starts the protective mechanism.

It tries to lower energy needs. The water in your body apart from keeping you hydrated also helps in regulating the body temperature. However, as soon as you lower the calorie intake the body starts dumping the water to compensate for the energy deficit. But, there is nothing to worry as this is a temporary phenomenon and the water levels in your body would be back soon.

When you begin fasting your body also starts cleaning itself of the toxins and that also causes frequent urination. As long as you are not feeling any discomfort or the trips haven't increased a lot, it is not something that should worry you much.

You should keep drinking lots of water to compensate for the loss. If hypertension or other such medical issues are not there, you should even try having water with a pinch of sea salt. It helps in replenishing the loss of minerals that occurs due to excessive urination.

Binge Eating:

Once the fast is over, there are those who start eating and can't stop. With normal eating, they were able to control their appetite just fine, but with extended periods of not eating, their appetite seems insatiable. The inability to control appetite is a problem in itself. If the binge eating continues, the calories taken replace what has just been lost during the fast, and no weight will be lost despite all the effort. Worse still, more calories will be consumed than those lost, adding even more body fat.

Hyper-acidity:

The stomach contains acids which aid digestion. In the absence of food, you may feel stinging heartburn that could extend to the throat area. It is possible to experience heartburn during fasting that you previously did not experience at all.

Disrupted Sleep:

There are those who cannot sleep when hungry. Think about it; even in normal days, when you can sleep, you most probably end up in the kitchen taking a snack. A full stomach does encourage sleep, as all the energy is directed towards digesting the meal. You may have noticed that when you take a heavy lunch, you spend the afternoon feeling drowsy. An empty stomach could result in poor sleep, and you'll then spend the following day sleepy and fatigued.

Low Energy and Irritability:

Depending on how you are eating, your body may also be growing used to consuming fat as a fuel source rather than carbohydrates. So, in addition of losing its primary energy source, it is also have to switch how it consumes energy and where it comes from. This can lead to lowered energy for a while. The best thing to do during this time is to relax and keep your days as free as possible. Do things that exert the least amount of energy. If you are someone who regularly exercises and works out, reducing the amount that you work out or switching to a more relaxed workout like yoga can help you during the transition period.

In addition to feeling low energy, you may also feel irritability. Irritability is often caused by low energy and hunger. This may be frustrating early on as your body begins to adjust. Again, take it easy, reduce the amount of stress that you have in your daily life if possible, and give yourself time to adjust. Once you are used to your new eating habits the irritability will subside and your energy levels will pick up once again.

One common issue that people can have while beginning the fasting routine is a feeling of irritability. It isn't a permanent phenomenon and occurs only due to the fact that your blood sugar levels may fluctuate in the beginning. We have already discussed that your body may experience low blood sugar levels for extended periods and that is not a very bad thing if you are not suffering from some chronic problem like diabetes. However, low blood sugar can cause irritability as the body is frantically looking for energy.

This is the stage where even your body is learning through the transition phase. It is making the switch to the fat fuel when it doesn't want to. This is a temporary phenomenon that wouldn't last very long.

Heartburn, Bloating, and Constipation:
Heartburn and bloating are common issues that you may face when you begin fasting. The reasons for bloating are simple, your gut keeps releasing the digestive juices at regular intervals but doesn't get anything to digest that causes the problem. However, this is a very temporary phenomenon as your gut would easily adjust to your new eating schedules and the problem would subside.

The heartburns are also part of the same process but they cause the most discomfort. The good thing is that they wouldn't last long. As soon as the release of digestive juices gets timed, bloating and heartburn would subside.

Constipation, on the other hand, can be a problem for many. The main reason for constipation isn't fasting but intake of improper food. It is a fact that your food intake may reduce when you begin intermittent fasting as your number of meals go down. However, if you don't include high fiber food items in your meals, your gut wouldn't have much to process. This can cause constipation that may trouble you a lot. The best way to avoid is to have fiber-rich food. Increase the salads and fiber-rich food in your meals and you would face no such issue. The important thing to remember is that you need to understand the problems you are facing and try to find the solution. Don't stick to a particular thing but try to find your best in the routine.

Intermittent fasting may become a big change in your life. You will have to make a few adjustments to welcome this change. It would be easy for you and even beneficial if you start making some adjustment to accommodate them. Don't be stubborn or a stickler for rules. Try to find your rhythm and flow with it.

Chapter 6: Tips and Tricks To Follow Correctly

Do you know what a fasting regime and New Year resolutions have in common? They start out great for a couple of months. First going to the second month; doing well. The third month; some hitches here and there. By the 6th or 7th month, some people have a problem remembering what their resolutions were in the first place. In this case, some will not remember their proposed fasting plans.

If you have fallen by the wayside, you'll be relieved to know you're not alone. Even the most enthusiastic fitness guru struggles with staying on course. If you have already missed a few steps, you can start all over again and get it right this time.

Sample these tips which will help you stay motivated:

Get an Accountability Partner

Having someone alongside you with similar goals can keep you on course. With the internet, your accountability partner can even be in another continent. The point here is that you're answerable to someone. You know what being answerable does to you? It makes you do things even when you don't feel like. Like when you don't feel like getting up and going to work, but you remember you have a boss to answer to, and you jump out of bed. The accountability partner for your fasting journey maybe your peer, but questions will still be asked. This also comes with a level of competition. If your partner can fast for 24 hours, or manage on a certain number of calories, why can't you? And who lost more pounds this week? You definitely don't want to be the one trailing, at least not every time. This accountability/competition relationship will ensure that you stay on track when you've have otherwise fallen off the radar. In fact, it is possible to achieve more with an accountability partner as opposed to a mentor. A mentor strikes an imposing figure, sort of talking down at you from a high horse. Accountability partners are at your level, demanding of you the much they demand of themselves.

Keep Informed

How much do you know about intermittent fasting? The more you know, the easier it will be for you to go through the process. Read blogs and watch videos to see what other women, and indeed men have to say about the fast. You'll realize that you're not alone in the issues you're experiencing.

This will also help you keep your expectations realistic. When it comes to weight loss, women can be impatient. A few days on a diet and you're already in front of the mirror looking for changes. Don't worry; we've all been there! You know by now that intermittent fasting is a way to lose weight fast; but how fast is fast? Getting the right information from those who have gone through the fast will let you know what to expect, and you'll be better prepared to deal with the process.

Set Goals with Rewards

Setting milestones with some goodies attached to them will keep you going even when your body and mind tells you otherwise. Keep in mind that the reward, in this case, is not food related.

Why can't you treat your sweet tooth as a reward? Well, to begin with, what you'd be saying to your mind is that the healthy foods you're eating are a punishment of sort, and only after eating them will you get some 'good' food.

Secondly, if you indulge in sugary and fatty treats, you'll only roll back on the gains already made. We don't want any of that, do we?

Your goal here is mainly weight loss, among other health gains. Once you've reached a goal of losing a certain number of pounds in a set time, you can treat yourself with a shopping trip for new clothes. Enjoy fitting in clothes that you would not have worn previously. As you look at yourself in the mirror and admire the new you, you'll be even more motivated to work towards your next goal.

Concentrate on Positive Feelings

How do you feel after shedding some pounds? I'm sure you're enjoying fitting into a smaller size of outfits, looking more presentable, feeling confident, being physically active without straining and so on.

Let these feelings color your day. Every time a thought crops up on how hungry you are, or how many foods you can no longer eat, remind yourself how dashing you look in that new dress. If you catch yourself staring at the clock gloomily counting how many more hours you have left on your fast, remind yourself that you can now make work presentations more confidently, presenting a positive body image.

Every time a negative feeling lingers, counter it with a positive thought and watch your energy revive.

64

Healthy-Eating Mind

Reprogram your mind to look at intermittent fasting, and indeed healthy eating as a whole as a positive lifestyle and not retribution. We're so accustomed to this random lifestyle where we eat what we want when we want it; that anything short of that feels like a punishment. Living healthy is choosing to be kind to your body, and knowing that it will remit the kindness right back. Think of your body for a moment as a separate entity from yourself. How would it feel when constantly being fed on the wrong foods that bring you terrible effects? How would it feel to constantly be fed on too much food and you have to strain to digest? If your body could speak, it could possibly ask these questions.

Feed it on the right foods, because it is the right thing to do. Give it just the right amount, without overloading it with unnecessary carbs, sugar, and fats. And give it a break from all the digesting work occasionally, who does not like a good rest?

Visualize the Future

Just picture how your future will turn out if you keep living this healthy lifestyle. You'll be disease-free, active, radiant and energetic. You'll improve your longevity, enjoying a longer, fuller life.

What's the other side of the coin? A life full of diseases. I'm sure you know such people, maybe even in your family, whose lives have been dimmed by disease. They're no longer able to do the things they enjoy. Their activity level is largely reduced if not cut off altogether. They are dependent on others to assist them even with minor roles. They carry medicine wherever they go. Isn't the idea of such a life horrifying, especially in a case where different choices were all was needed for a different turnout?

Choosing health is choosing life. If you still have the chance, this is an opportunity that you have to embrace. You work so hard to ensure your later days will see you age gracefully, do not let unhealthy living take this dream away from you.

Join a Community of Like Minds

Thank God for the internet; we can now form groups with people of similar interests even from different continents. Search the internet for women in intermittent fasting, and you should be able to find such groups. You can then exchange messages, photos, and videos of your progress. With a group also comes competition. We agree our bodies are different, but you definitely don't want to be the one trailing the lot by losing the least weight. That only helps you stay consistent. Share experiences, tips, goals, recipes, survival tactics and so on. Alone you can get discouraged and quit, but such a 'healthy living family' will not let you fall by the wayside.

Take Help of Positive Affirmations

Positive affirmations are very inspiring. They fill us with positive energy and help in clearing away negative thoughts. You can read positive affirmations, listen to them on the internet or recite them loudly. They help in every way. Positive affirmations keep your mind clear and give you the energy to sail through the bad times. They don't take much of your time and you also don't have to remain dependent on others. Taking help of positive affirmations is a great way to remain motivated.

Share Your Goals with Your Family and Friends

Sharing such things with others is always difficult. There is always the fear of being judged on the results. However, there are always some people in everyone's life who don't judge. It can be your parents, partner, siblings, or close friends. Share your goals with them and the problems you are facing in the way. Discuss with them the ways to get out of the problems. They can give you suggestions or at least lend their ears. Even letting it off your chest is also a great relief most of the times.

You will always have an assurance that there are people who really understand your efforts and are supporting you in them. It is not necessary that you disclose your goals to everyone but sharing it with some of your very close people is always a good idea.

Professional Help

Obesity is not a rare problem these days. In fact, it is one of the most common ailments faced by people. Therefore, you can also get several professionals with whom you can discuss your problems and progress. You can consult your doctor and periodically discuss your progress. This serves two purposes. First, there will be a professional to guide you about the progress. You will get professional opinions on time about the problems you face on your way. You can get tips on nutrition and also advice about the ways to improve the progress.

Support Groups

It is a cost-effective way to get help. Support groups can emerge as pillars of strength. There are many people suffering from the same problems. They are also going through the same trials and tribulations. They can prove to be a great help in case you need moral or mental support. Most of the people in support groups are facing similar problems and hence your problems can be common. You can get the tips that worked for them. Such support groups can be of great help.

Keep the Atmosphere at Your Home Conducive

Most of the time, the atmosphere around us makes our efforts difficult. For instance, if your fridge is full of carbonated beverages, fast food snacks and munchies, it would be difficult to control the urge to eat. If people in your home are casually eating things all the time, you would start feeling punished and left out. It is important that you explain your goals and make arrangements so that the process gets simpler and not difficult. It is important that you clear your fridge. If it is shared by others then you should limit your access to the fridge. Your kitchen should be stacked with healthy things and junk food should be removed so that you don't get tempted and eat it.

Remove all kinds of sweets and chocolates from your home. They are irresistible and can break your will in your weak moments.

By thinking of losing weight you have already cleared the first hurdle. You only need to become more conscious of your choices to succeed in your efforts.

Chapter 7: What Foods & Liquids Do

When you go about your first round of intermittent fasting, you'll need to know what to avoid and what to keep close at hand.

When it comes to foods, the best things to have around <u>are</u>:

All Legumes and Beans – good carbs can help lower body weight without planned calorie restriction

Anything high in protein – helpful in keeping your energy levels up in your efforts as a whole, even when you're in a period of fasting

Anything with the herbs cayenne pepper, psyllium, or dried/crushed dandelion – they'll contribute to weight loss without sacrificing calories or effort

Avocado – a high-, good-calorie fruit that has a lot of healthy fats

Berries – often high in antioxidants and vitamin C as well as flavonoids for weight loss

Cruciferous Vegetables – broccoli, cauliflower, brussel sprouts, and more are incredibly high in fiber, which you'll definitely want to keep constipation at bay with IF

Eggs – high in protein and great for building muscle during IF periods

Nuts & Grains – sources of healthy fats and essential fiber

Potatoes – when prepared in healthy ways, they satiate hunger well and help with weight loss

Wild-Caught Fish – high in healthy fats while providing protein and vitamin D for your brain

When it comes to liquids, some of it is pretty self-explanatory:

- *Water* - It's always good for you! It will help keep you hydrated, it will provide relief with headaches or light headedness or fatigue, and it clears out your system in the initial detox period.

Try adding a squeeze of lemon, some cucumber or strawberry slices, or a couple of sprigs of mint, lavender, or basil to give your water some flavor if you're not enthused with the taste of it plain.

If you need something else to drink, you can seek out:

- *Probiotic drinks like kefir or kombucha*

You can even look for probiotic foods such *as sauerkraut, kimchi, miso, pickles, yogurt, tempeh*, and more!

- *Probiotics* work amazingly well at healing your gut especially in times of intense transition, as with the start of intermittent fasting.

- *Black coffee,* whenever possible, in moderation

Sweeteners and milk aren't productive for your fasting and weight loss goals.

- Heated or chilled *vegetables* or bone broths

- *Teas* of any kind

- *Apple cider vinegar* shots

Instead, try water or other drinks with ACV mixed in.

<u>Drinks to avoid</u> would be:

- *Regular soda*

- *Diet soda*

- *Alcohol* of any kind

- *High-sugar coconut and almond drinks*

- *i.e. coconut water, coconut milk, almond milk, etc.*

- *Anything with artificial sweetener* will shock your insulin levels into imbalance with your blood sugar later on

Go for the low-sugar or unsweetened milk alternative if it's available.

Focus on Healthy Food

The human body needs macronutrients, minerals, and vitamins to function properly. All of them can be found in food, but unfortunately, the food available nowadays is not very consistent in nutrients. Most of the food we eat today is processed, and the more processed food is, the unhealthier and less consistent in nutrients. Also, processed food is rich in carbs, a macronutrient which can cause terrible effects to the human body. In fact, food has killed more people over the last few decades than drugs, alcohol, and cigarettes put together. Around 70% of the diseases known today are caused by food. You are probably asking yourself why this happens. The answer lies with processed foods and carbs, as they are the roots of all these problems. Carbs can be split into sugar and starch, and sugar really needs no introduction, as it's perhaps the most harmful substance ever to be consumed by humans. Without any doubt, food was a lot healthier 100 years ago, and there weren't so many cases of obesity and diabetes (both caused by an excess of carbs). The problem with sugar is that we consume it voluntarily and even feed it to our children. This kind of food causes addiction, as you will not feel satiety for a long time (in fact, you will feel hungry sooner), it won't cover the body's nutritional needs and you will crave some more carbs very soon. Those carbs contain glucose, which can be used by the body to generate energy, but this energy is produced only through physical exercise. The glucose doesn't get consumed and instead gets stored in your blood, raising your insulin and blood sugar levels. This is one step closer to diabetes, so this is how it all gets started.

Most of the food we consume today is processed and even what it claims to be natural is not organic. Before being able to process food, the most processed food you can dream of was bread, but the recipe was pretty simplistic, so different than the bread we are consuming today. Food was cooked from natural ingredients, and it had great nutritional value. Also, the lifestyle was a lot more active, as there weren't too many means of transportation back then. When we think of natural food nowadays, it's simply very difficult to find organic food, as chemicals are used to grow fruits, vegetables or crops. Fertilizers are no longer natural (with high chemical content), and animals are being fed concentrated food to grow incredibly fast. The meat we are consuming comes from these animals, and if they are fed this kind of food, this will affect us. Processing food is all about adding extra value to the product, otherwise, companies operating in this domain can't seem to find a way to increase their profits. It's fair to say that for the sake of profits, food processing companies are literally making poison to be consumed by the people. Everything which is packed and has more ingredients (many of them being chemicals you can't even pronounce) is processed food. This type of food is promoted by supermarkets and fast-food restaurants, as it fits perfectly with the current way of life. Finding healthy food is becoming a challenge nowadays, especially for the people who want to cut down on carbs. You are probably wondering what exactly you can eat in order to stay away from carbs.

Intermittent fasting is a procedure of self-discipline, in which you impose on yourself a strict set of rules and eat only within the designated feeding window. For most of the programs, there is no mention of what you can eat. However, this doesn't mean that you can stuff yourself with junk food. Healthy food can improve the results of this program, and there are a few options when it comes to healthy diets. You can consider a keto diet, a Mediterranean diet or an alkaline diet, and they all involve consuming plenty of vegetables and less meat. Most of them are LCHF (low carb high fat) diets, but the protein intake may vary from one diet to another. This diet traces its roots from the living habits of the people living in the Mediterranean basin, so it doesn't mean just Italian cuisine. But be careful, as this diet doesn't include pizza and it doesn't focus on

74

pasta. This kind of diet has its very own food pyramid, based on how frequent you should try that food type.

If the standard food pyramid has **6 different levels**:

1) *Vegetables, salad, fruits*

2) *Bread, whole-grain cereals, pasta, potatoes, and rice* - the food category richest in carbs

3) *Milk, yogurt and cheese*

4) *Meat, poultry, fish, eggs, beans, and nuts*

5) *Oils, spread, and fats*

6) *Sweets, snacks, soft drinks, juices* - basically food and drinks with very high levels of sugar and salt

The Mediterranean diet has it figured differently, as you can see below:

1) The base of the pyramid is represented by the *physical activity*, as this is a lifestyle for people living in the Mediterranean region.

2) The second level of the pyramid includes different types of food like *fruits, vegetables, beans, nuts, olive oil, seeds and legumes, herbs and spices, but also grains* (with a focus on whole grains). Most of the foods on this level should be consumed on a daily basis.

3) The third level of the pyramid is represented by *seafood and fish*, which should be consumed approximately twice a week.

4) The next level features poultry, *cheese, yogurt, and eggs.*

5) The last level of the pyramid is represented by *meat and sweets.*

The logic behind this pyramid is the same as with the standard food pyramid, the more necessary the food type is, the lower is on the pyramid. The Mediterranean diet includes a plethora of food types to choose from, all healthy, delicious and nutritious. Therefore, it's probably the most complete meal plan you can associate with intermittent fasting. You can eat fish, seafood, meat, chicken, turkey, but most of all, you will need to consume veggies, fruits, seeds, nuts, dairy products, and also olive oil. This diet focuses on healthy unsaturated fats, so it's exactly what the body needs for the IF lifestyle, as it can bring your body into ketosis (the metabolic state when ketones are multiplying to break down the fat tissue).

Some of the main features of the Mediterranean diet <u>are</u>:

- Focus on the consumption of *fruits, nuts, veggies, legumes, and whole grains*

- There is also a high emphasis on consuming healthy fats from *canola or olive oil*

- <u>Forget</u> about the use of salt to flavor your food, as this diet encourages the use of herbs and spices

- <u>Less red meat</u> (<u>pork or beef</u>) and more *fish or chicken/turkey*

- You can even *drink red wine* <u>in moderate quantities</u>

It doesn't sound like a diet at all, as there are so many types of food accepted. It's more of a lifestyle than a meal plan. If a standard diet is something you need to stick to for a few weeks, the Mediterranean diet is the meal plan that you have to stick to for the rest of your life. It can include all 3 meals of the day, but you can also have snacks or desserts. It sounds too good to be true? Well, this is what the Mediterranean diet is, and it can work wonders on you if you combine it with intermittent fasting and working out. But, that's not all! By now you already know the benefits of intermittent fasting. How about adding some more benefits by following this type of diet? If you want stronger bones, lower risk of frailty, lung disease or heart disease, and even to ward off depression, then you definitely need to try this diet.

Since this meal plan is diversified, you don't have to make radical changes in your refrigerator, as you are probably already consuming some of the foods mentioned here. However, at least when it comes to veggies, legumes, and fruits, you will need to eat them fresh, so frequent shopping may be required.

You need to know that the ingredients of the Mediterranean diet are structured into **11 categories**, as you can see below:

1) *Vegetables* are one of the most important categories included in this meal plan and you can consume them frozen or fresh. In the frozen veggies group there can be included peas, green beans, spinach or others. In terms of fresh vegetables, you can buy tomatoes, cucumbers, peppers, onions, okra, green beans, zucchini, garlic, peas, cauliflower, mushrooms,

broccoli, potatoes, peas, carrots, celery leaves, cabbage, spinach, beets, or romaine lettuce.

2) The *fruits* you need to include in your shopping list are peaches, pears, figs, apricots, apples, oranges, tangerines, lemons, cherries, and watermelon.

3) You can't have a Mediterranean diet without some *high-fat dairy products*. Milk (whether is whole or semi-skimmed) is no longer considered a good option, as it also has a higher concentration of carbs. You can buy instead sheep's milk yogurt, Greek yogurt, feta cheese, ricotta (or other types of fresh cheese), mozzarella, groviera, and mizithra.

4) This diet doesn't focus too much on *meat or poultry,* but you can still eat them twice a week. Your shopping list will need to include chicken (whether you prefer it whole, breasts or thighs), pork, ground beef, and veal. This is where you can get most of your proteins from, but still, you need to keep the protein intake at a low level.

5) Can you imagine a Mediterranean diet without *fish or seafood?* This food is a must in this meal plan, although you can only have it twice a week. So, you will need to buy salmon, tuna, cod, sardines, anchovies, shrimp, octopus or calamari. You can eat some of them fresh or canned.

6) Although you don't have to abuse them, your shopping list should definitely include *bread or pasta.* If they are made from whole grains are even better, as they are the right choice in this case. Try to avoid the unnecessary consumption of pastry, like having bagels, pretzels or croissants with your coffee. You can eat and buy instead whole grains

bread, paximadi (barley rusks), breadsticks (also made from whole grains), pita bread, phyllo, pasta, rice, egg pasta, bulgur, and couscous.

7) Your shopping list must include *healthy fats and nuts*. Olive oil should be consumed on a daily basis, so you need to have it in your household. Also, in terms of nuts, it's recommended that you buy tahini, almonds, walnuts, pine nuts, pistachios, and sesame seeds.

8) *Beans* are an important part of this diet, so you definitely need to buy lentils, white beans chickpeas, and fava.

9) *Pantry items* are the miscellaneous part of this meal plan. In this group, you can include olives, canned tomatoes, tomato paste, sun-dried tomatoes, capers, herbal tea, honey, balsamic or red wine vinegar and wine (preferably red).

10) As mentioned above, *herbs and spices* are used for flavoring your food. As this diet involves a lot of home cooking, having plenty of spices and herbs can make a difference. That's why your shopping list must include herbs and spices like oregano, mint, dill, parsley, cumin, basil, sea salt, black pepper, cinnamon, sea salt and all kind of spices.

11) You definitely need to buy some *greens*, like chicory, dandelion, beet greens and amaranth and include them in your meal plan.

Calories Management

The first and perhaps one of the most important parts of successfully eating the intermittent fasting diet without any serious side effects is maintaining a proper calorie count each day. Having a smaller eating window can make this more challenging, so it is important that you are eating properly during these windows.

If you begin eating the intermittent fasting diet and do not receive enough calories, the impacts that you might experience could be quite negative. In addition to experiencing things like excessive hunger and headaches, you may also begin experiencing excessive weight loss. Weight loss on the intermittent fasting diet is a great side effect, but not if it is happening because you are quite literally starving.

It is important that you discover what the healthy calorie intake is for your age and weight range. Then, make sure that you are incorporating that caloric intake into your eating window. This may mean that during your eating window you are eating fairly consistently in order to get in enough calories to remain healthy. Focus on eating calorie-dense foods that are high in nutrition, such as meats and vegetables, to get your intake up. This will ensure that you stay well-nourished and that you do not begin losing weight as a result of starvation.

Lowered Carbs Intake:
Many people who realize that they need to increase their calorie intake in a short amount of time may look towards pasta and other carbs for their caloric value. Unfortunately, pasta and other carbohydrates are not ideal when it comes to using the intermittent fasting diet. They lack a rich nutritional value and are more likely to increase weight gain, elevate blood sugars, and cause bloating and constipation, especially if they are a primary food that you consume to attempt to reach your caloric intake through carbs.

In addition to their ability to spike your blood sugars, carbs also cause other side effects that can make intermittent fasting more challenging. For example, you might find that you are irritable and more tired when you consume a high level of carbs each day. You might also find that you struggle concentrating and that getting through your fasting cycles is more of a challenge. You can avoid these side effects by reducing carbs in your diet.

When you are intermittently fasting, a good idea is to avoid high carb intake altogether. Eating a low carb or ketogenic diet can support you in getting all of the nutrition that you need without consuming carbohydrates as a filler. This will not only support you in avoiding the unwanted side effects but will also ensure that you are gaining the maximum value of your diet. Lowering your carbohydrates will actually increase the level of ketones in your body, making it even easier for you to experience increased energy, weight loss, and muscle gain.

Increased Healthy Fats:

Since the intermittent diet increases ketones in your body, you want to increase healthy fats in your diet. Ketones are responsible for supporting your body in using fat as a fuel instead of sugars. This means that you need to have a healthy amount of fats for the ketones to effectively work on your body. This might seem counterintuitive since you want to burn fats, but it is actually essential. You need to provide your body with enough fuel to help it maintain itself and stay functioning and healthy.

Increasing your intake of healthy fats throughout your eating windows can support your body in having plenty of fats to produce energy from. It

81

is important that you choose healthy fats for this, as this will keep your fuel clean and effective. Filling up on unhealthy fats can be dangerous as it can actually have a negative impact on heart and blood health. Fats like the ones you get from avocado oil and coconut oil, nuts and seeds, fish, and cheeses can support you in maintaining your energy and staying healthy while eating the intermittent fasting diet. I have included a list of healthy fats below to give you an idea of what to look for and where to start.

Avoiding Sugary and Starchy Foods:
Sugary and starchy foods should be avoided in any diet. They can reduce metabolic efficiency and cause blood sugar spikes. When you are intermittently fasting, avoiding these types of foods can help you maintain your overall health. It can also support you in reducing negative side effects during your fasting cycles.

Ideally, you want to avoid sugars in any variety. This means that you should lower the amount of processed sugars and sweets that you eat, as well as reduce the amount of fruit you eat. If you are going to eat something sweet, however, opt for fruits over processed sugars. This will ensure that you are maintaining healthy blood sugar levels. This will also help your body continue using ketones and fat as fuel instead of sugar and carbs. In the end, you will get better results from your diet.

Starches can also break down and become sugars in the body, so it is important to avoid these, too. This means avoiding things like potatoes, corn, peas, rice, and beans. That way, your body can continue operating optimally and you get the best results from your diet.

Chapter 8: Hormonal Regulation And How Its Impacted By Intermittent Fasting

Hormonal regulation is a significant benefit of intermittent fasting. Women, in particular benefit from the effects of fasting, especially when it involves stabilizing certain hormones while increasing or decreasing other hormones. There are several ways in which intermittent can regulate hormone production. One of the most significant advantages of fasting is the reversal of insulin resistance. When the body sugar levels rise consistently, this increases glucose, and creates a resistance to insulin. Periods of fasting, both short and long terms, help the body regain the normal, healthy level of sensitivity towards insulin. This has the effect of regulating insulin, which is a hormone, and helps prevent to onset of type 2 diabetes. Growth hormones are important for helping the body burn fat and build muscle. During periods of intermittent fasting, growth hormones increase significantly, which helps accelerate weight loss and build muscle mass.

How Intermittent Fasting Affects Women Differently Than Men

Women of all ages benefit from intermittent fasting, from early 20s, through perimenopause, menopause and into senior years. There are emerging studies and results that show a different impact on women and men, when it comes to the impact of intermittent fasting. One of the major reasons for this difference is how women's bodies are more adapted to storing fat, which is significantly changed once weight loss begins during fasting. Low to zero calorie intake during a fast can cause side effects in some women, such as cramps and changes in menstruation. This can occur with prolonged fasting, though most side effects or discomfort associated with cessation of food is temporary, for both men and women.

The **advantages** of intermittent fasting for women are significant, and are often directly connected to hormones and their production:

- Lower insulin levels in women keep blood sugar low on a consistent basis. This occurs after only a few weeks of regular intermittent fasting. This seems to remain consistent in the long term, with overall changes in insulin at normal levels.

- Inflammation is reduced, and specifically inflammation and weight gain associated with chronic conditions showed significant improvement over time. As chronic inflammation can cause weight gain, this also results in weight maintenance, in addition to weight loss.

- Depression affects a lot of people, which can trigger other habits, such as overeating and not getting regular exercise. One study noted that after eight weeks of intermittent fasting, there was a noticeable decline in depression. This affects a lot of women during different stages of life: post-partum, perimenopause, and during menstrual cycles. While it is not advised to practice intermittent fasting during pregnancy or while breastfeeding,

85

eating healthy, nutritious meals is a good way to get everything you need, until you are ready to start a fasting method.

- Women more than men, lose bone mass as they age. Preserving muscle mass is of utmost importance at all stages in life, though more so in advanced age. Restricting calories through fasting, rather than calorie restricted diets that do not include fasts in the plan, show a better retention of muscle mass. This helps the body break down fat and aids in weight loss.

While all fasting methods are beneficial for women, some studies indicate that regular use of certain fasting programs are ideal:

- *24-hour fasting, done twice each week*

- *16:8 and 18:6 fasting methods*

- *5:2 fasting*

IF & the Female Body

Since intermittent fasting is not so much a diet as it is an altered pattern in eating times and frequency, its relationship with the female body is not the same as the standard diet's relationship would be. In fact, it's not necessarily supportive for females to practice a strict diet while intermittent fasting, for the combination of the two, can work serious havoc on the female body itself.

To counteract any curious side-effects of IF on your physical and mental states, you can try and make sure to eat as nutritious a selection of food as you can, whenever possible. Furthermore, you can try not to *over*exert yourself through exercise, especially since you're altering your food and nutrition intake significantly. Also, you can ensure that you're not forcing yourself to engage in IF if you're ill, suffering from an infection, or struggling with a chronic disorder of some kind. Finally, if your body is exhausted due to work or struggles with anxiety (or otherwise), you might not want to put yourself through additional stress with a new pattern of eating.

The most important thing to do as you begin to engage with intermittent fasting as a female-bodied person is to make sure you're as connected to (and introspective of) your body as you can be, as often as you're able to be. The more you know your body and its tendencies (i.e. the frequency of your period, your tendencies with metabolism, your fat storage areas, your most common moods, your emotional crutches, etc.), the more successful your experiences with intermittent fasting can be.

Physical Effects of IF for Women

While the general effects of intermittent fasting include increased energy overall, clearer cognition and memory, improved immunity, slowed aging process, better heart health, increased insulin sensitivity, and more, are some of the physical effects for women deserve a little more detail in specific.

For women, it **includes**:

-   Lowered blood pressure in about two months or less, lowered cholesterol by ¼ the original toxic amount, better blood sugar control, decreased likelihood for type 2 diabetes, lowered chances of cancer, potential for increased muscle mass (with the ability to preserve it longer!), increased lifespan by up to 50 years, and increased awareness of internal bodily processes in general.

- After a few months of intermittent fasting practice, you're sure to feel that your senses are somewhat heightened compared to how they were before, that your body works better and smoother than ever, that your weight melts off like wax from a candle, and that your mind and cognition are clearer than ever before.

- Some physical effects function almost like warning signs for the woman practicing IF, too. If you experience poorer skin conditions, complete insomnia, loss of hair, excessive or shocking decrease in muscle mass, loss of period entirely, heart arrhythmia, or increased inflammations (whether internally or externally), you'll definitely want to consider altering your process, stopping the IF for a while, or visiting a nearby doctor for advice.

Using IF to Help with Periods, Fertility, and Metabolism

If you struggle monthly through painful periods; if you know you don't want to have children and you're not concerned about future fertility; or if you want to kick-start your metabolism to help yourself lose weight, all you have to do is start intermittently fasting without any concern whatsoever. If you're looking for hard and fast changes for your harsh menses, your fertility, or your weight issues, work your way up to fasting a few days a week, and you're sure to see the side-effects you seek played out within a month or two.

If you're interested in getting help with painful periods without substantial effects on your future fertility, simply make sure to get enough fat in your diet and supplemental estrogen (which you can find over the counter in a variety of forms). By making sure to consume enough healthy fat and by not restricting your caloric intake too much, you can use intermittent fasting to ease difficult menses without it having too much effect on your metabolism at the moment, and with it having hardly any effect on your fertility later on.

If you want the metabolism boost without effect on your periods or fertility, here's what you can do. Make sure you're eating enough healthy fats, but restrict caloric intake slightly, not too much though, mind you! You don't want to hurt those hunger hormones or inhibit your ability to ovulate and have a healthy period!

For these reasons, you should make sure *not* to intentionally or fastidiously "diet" while you're intermittently fasting but seeing as how you *do* want to lose weight and kick-start that metabolism, you can do *something* to help your body remember not to hang onto too much excess! That "*something*" that works so well is two-part: (1) once you define your method, keep to its timing strictly and; (2) when you have your meals, don't overindulge, binge, or gorge yourself; allow your caloric intake to be limited, but only slightly, as you work with IF.

Chapter 9: Intermittent Fasting For Weight Loss

Learn About Your Natural Eating Pattern

The first step towards any change in diet is *awareness*. Start paying attention to what you're eating and begin being conscious of your dietary choices.

The best way to keep track of them is to write them down in a small notebook. Carry a pen and paper or make notes in an app on your phone or tablet about when and what you eat. Most people are shocked by how much they eat in a day. Identifying personal eating patterns and the types of foods preferred is the appropriate place to start when embarking on intermittent fasting.

Create a food journal or log (you will find a link in bonus section to get a copy of a free printable food journal) that includes **the following items**:

- *Log the Date and day of the week:* Note whether it's morning, noon, or night. You'll have to be time-specific when you start fasting.

- *What are all the foods and drinks consumed:* List the types, amounts, and whether you added calories through use of condiments, butter, sugar, *etc.* Beverages count, so make note of them too. Keep notes on what you add to your beverages, such as sugar or honey as a sweetener. This will be important later.

- *Portion sizes:* Estimates of the volume, weight or number of items works just fine. If you prefer to measure, that's great as well. The point is to get a sense of quantity.

- *The location of your meals:* Take notes of where you are at mealtimes. Are you in a car, at a desk, or on a couch? Are you eating alone or with other people?

- *What is your activity level while eating:* Pay attention to what you are focused on as you're eating food. Are you browsing the internet or checking Instagram, or simply talking with friends?

- *How are you feeling:* What are your emotions? Are you happy, excited, depressed, stressed, anxious, or content? Our emotions can direct our eating choices, and conversely, eating can inspire emotions. Pay particular attention to increases in eating based on emotional situations.

To make your food journal valuable, be open and honest. Take the time to note every bite of food eaten and beverage you drink. If you don't log everything, you won't have an accurate picture of your dietary habits. For the most accurate results, try to record your food intake within 15 minutes of the time you eat.

Intermittent Fasting and Exercise

Myths still exist that caution people away from getting involved in any type of exercise program or physical training during periods of intermittent fasting. Although it's true that your body will not perform well for an extended period of time on empty, but true intermittent

91

fasting is not about complete deprivation. It is periodic, scheduled time away from food that lasts for mere hours.

As long as you follow the correct methods for intermittent fasting and eat right during your window of nutritional opportunity, you can use exercise routines to increase the power output of your body. Running lean means a more efficient firing of your internal engine.

Transition Slowly

Think of your first month of intermittent fasting as an experiment, rather than a difficult task you must do in order to be healthy. Just relax and break it down into small, manageable tasks you know you can accomplish. When you're ready, consider increasing the number of days in the week that you fast for 14-hours, or consider fasting longer on the days of the week you choose to fast. See below for an example of how to build on the plan described above by adding a *15-hour fasting period* to your schedule.

Learn to Listen to Your Body

Observe how your body responds and think about anything that comes up. The goal is learning from this process and finding a way to do it that works for you. If you start to feel hunger cravings or like you are depriving yourself without cause, return to the reasons why you decided to try intermittent fasting and revisit the benefits. It's a good idea to avoid snacks. Keep this principle at the front of your mind as you begin exploring how to incorporate intermittent fasting into your life. The goal is to eat consciously and that often means breaking old eating habits that no longer serve us.

Symptoms You Should Watch for

If you don't feel well, do not delay breakfast, even if it is the first time you are trying intermittent fasting. If you skipped dinner the night before, and wake up not feeling well, eat something simple. If you need to eat breakfast at 7 am, give yourself permission to do so this time. It's not a problem. That's 12-hours out of 24, and it's a fine place to start. All you had to do was get through the tough time after dinner, go to bed, and wake up. It's ideal to have an open and honest discussion with your physician before embarking on the intermittent fasting diet. You should always heed their advice if you have any underlying medical conditions or take prescription medications. Certain medicines can interfere with the effectiveness of this diet regime. And, most importantly, if you are ill, or begin to feel sick, stop fasting.

Chapter 10: Intermittent Fasting And Other Diets

There are many different ways to construct your diet. All the fads that come and go may seem suitable for a week or two but often fall short on results and fulfillment. When seeking to improve your diet look to time-tested meal plans, find the ones based on distinct cultures or with a rich history of being locally sourced. You can make your choices for your diet, you can have some days that are vegetarian and some days that are not, there really are no official rules for diet except what you find to be fitting and what works for you. Be creative and open-minded in choosing meal plans.

We will now explore popular diets that also conform to the standards of an intermittent fasting routine. These diets are in no way the only paths to take when choosing a diet but we selected these diets to reflect ideal examples for intermittent fasting practices. We must keep in mind the importance of listening to our bodies and how they react to different diets. If you're unsure about a certain diet, simply test it out for a few days or weeks.

Let's look at **these diets** below:

Raw Food Diet

This diet is relatively self-explanatory. The guidelines are simple: eat only raw foods. Many people seeking to adhere to this diet gradually introduce raw foods into their usual diet until they feel comfortable with a completely raw diet. And when we say raw, that's strictly what we mean. These are uncooked and unprocessed foods. No dehydration or preservation but raw, fresh foods, often times not even seasoned with salt. While the nutritional value is not up for debate, the raw diet can be a bit limiting.

You will need consistent access to fresh foods and would typically find it tough to dine with friends who aren't adhering to a raw diet. This structure is probably the toughest to uphold with the least amount of options available.

A raw shopping list would look like this:

- *Nuts*

- *Seeds*

- *Fruits*

- *Vegetables*

- *Smoothies* and salads rule this diet

It is tough to fill yourself on raw foods successfully, not to mention it can be costly to supply because it is nothing but fresh foods from day to day.

This diet acts as a great way to cleanse and experiment with but rarely is it practiced for lifelong periods of time aside from a minority of people.

Paleo Diet

The paleo diet has seen very positive responses from weight lifting communities as well as those seeking a diet that is rich in cultural history. The paleo diet is based on what we now believe that our ancestors ate during hunter-gatherer eras. These were the times before agriculture saw plenty of meat being consumed as well as raw nuts, seeds, and berries. Some may even feel inclined to actually forage for the foods or hunt for their meat sources. Scientific studies show insight into these times, suggesting that our ancestors were very active and essentially maintained a mostly raw diet, and more interestingly, may have fasted during times of unsuccessful hunts or forages. There is a common misconception that prehistoric man ate nothing but meat. This is up for debate but the majority of experts suggest that the inconsistency of hunts and large tribe size would mean that less than half of the diet would consist of meat. This could vary greatly in different regions of the world and with the mysterious nature of our past, it is tough to accurately suggest how our ancestors lived. We can safely assume that they ate a diet high in protein and fiber, with very little caloric intake, here we see that this concept fits nicely into intermittent fasting practices.

While the paleo diet has varying philosophies person to person, the structure is pretty consistent. Although pinpointing the exact diet of past generations is an ill-fated task, we can give a loose guideline for what is today considered a paleo diet.

It is <u>as it follows</u>:

- *Lean meats and seafood*

- *Eggs*

- *Root vegetables*

- *Seeds*

- *Nuts*

- *Fruits*

- *Oils such as olive or coconut*

- *Herbs*

This is not a comprehensive list but a solid beginner's guide to starting to work with a paleo style diet. Keep in mind these ingredients would be wild foraged or trapped and hunted on the day of consumption. The fresher the ingredient, the closer to a legitimate paleo diet it is. There are also many foods avoided by adherents of the paleo diet. Consider that agriculture and farming wouldn't have existed, so many foods that are available and popular in our society today would not be accessible.

Some examples include:

- *Legumes*

- *Grains*

- *Dairy Products*

- *Processed oils*

- *Processed sweeteners*

- *Any processed or frozen food*

Whole Thirty Diet

Rising in popularity in recent years with the many diagnoses of celiac and other gluten intolerances, the whole thirty diet requires one to give up foods that are common allergies for many people. The idea that these foods are the cause of humans developing the allergies is at the heart of this diet. These foods are seen as undesirable for adherents of this diet. The practice of this diet itself asks that you do a thirty-day clean eating, cutting out these undesirable foods to see if you feel noticeably better due to an acute allergy to these common culprits.

The **foods** often <u>excluded</u> are as follows:

- *Peanuts*

- *Beans*

- *Grains, even gluten-free grains and other sources of gluten*

- *Shellfish*

- *Dairy*

- *Soy*

- *Nuts*

- *Seeds*

This list is certainly doesn't include every allergy causing food. If you suspect a food may be causing harmful reactions, cut it out during the clean eating cycle and see what happens. Upon gradually introducing these foods, you can take note of your body's reactions or lack thereof.

The whole thirty diet is a great diet for practicing awareness of our bodies. This diet can help us develop our skills and habits of listening to our bodies. By individually reintroducing foods after a type of cleanse, we can better learn how certain types of foods react when we ingest them. This makes the whole thirty diet ideal for preparing for intermittent fasting. Start the whole thirty diet about one month before a fasting week to ease into the IF mindset and prepare your body for dietary changes.

Vegetarian Diets

Plant-based diets are incredibly popular not only because of the internet and globalization but also many cultures have sustained a plant-based standard for millennia. Vegetarianism has seen incredible success in changing people's lives for the better, it is popular throughout the world, comprising over twenty percent of the entire population.

Many people are attracted to vegetarian diets to help counteract the western world's reliance on meat and animal products. Farming industries contribute to increase the world's pollution and deforestation problems so, with its health benefits and ecological awareness, vegetarianism acts a powerful diet to change your life on the individual level and your surrounding world.

Vegetarian guidelines are simple to follow. You essentially do not include any meat into your diet. This could mean many different things to many different people. Some people exclude meat itself but eat eggs and use animal-based broths. Other vegetarians exclude any animal products; so no dairy, broths, milk, or eggs. This more strict diet can borderline a vegan diet, but veganism tends to be stricter, promoting animal rights activism. Vegetarian diets usually include cheeses and dairy but it would be on only certain occasions.

The vegetarian diet is great for those who want a simple change to improve their diet, some people choose one day a week to each vegetarian; others explore the diet thoroughly, often taking in the eating habits for the rest of their lives.

Vegetarian ingredients would look like the following list:

- *Vegetables*

- *Fruits*

- *Nuts*

- *Seeds*

- *Berries*

- *Whole Grains*

- *Dairy*

- *Eggs*

- *Beans*

- *Soy or Tofu*

Vegan Diet

Adopting a vegan diet is similar to a vegetarian one, only vegans are strictly plant-based. It doesn't include any animal products at all. No dairy, no broths, no eggs, honey, and not even using make-up or wearing clothes made of animal products. We see here that this diet comes equipped with a philosophy. Animal activism is a crucial aspect of veganism. Many vegans protest the farming industry and even denounce domestication of animals. Social philosophy is not the intention of this book so we will leave it at that.

Vegan diets includes:

- *Strict no animal consumption*

- *Vegetables*

- *Fruits*

- *Whole Grains*

- *Nuts*

- *Seeds*

- *Berries*

- *Beans*

- *Soy or Tofu*

Mediterranean Diet

This diet has a rich history and cultural specificity, offering a lively timeline and time tested diet where the success is seen throughout all the cultures in the Mediterranean region. The positive and celebratory nature of the dining experience in these cultures is known throughout the world. This is why many travel to these regions simply to feast and enjoy life. This adheres to the theme throughout this book to build a relationship with food and eating that is positive and enjoyable. The people in the Mediterranean region are walking examples of the benefits of an enjoyable diet and food experience.

A Mediterranean shopping list may look similar to this:

- *Fruits*

- *Legumes*

- *Vegetables*

- *Fresh Fish*

- *Olive Oil*

The lean, low calorie and high-fat content of this diet make for a balanced diet that syncs well with an intermittent fasting routine. The relationship we build with our bodies should be enjoyable and shameless, pick a night to prepare a Mediterranean feast accompanied by a red wine from the region to break away from your usual routine.

Ketogenic Diet

We need to reiterate the dangers involved with inducing an intentional state of ketosis. If you are considering this type of diet, be sure to do your research and listen to your body. Let's discuss the ketogenic diet in more detail. Diets that adhere to a ketogenic structure are not typically practiced by beginners in the intermittent fasting communities. The diet is considered to be a more advanced structure than other popular diets. These diets are typically high in fat and very low in carbohydrate content. Whole grains and bread are avoided.

Some mandatory **foods** would be:

- *Eggs*

- *Avocados*

- *Fatty meats*

- *Fish*

The reasoning for this diet comes from the science of ketosis we touched on earlier in the book. By limiting caloric intake and lessening the quick energy we get from sugars and carbs, our bodies will burn stored fat cells as an alternative. Fat cells are cleaner and more efficient energy as well; this is why we see plenty of fats in a ketogenic diet. We can see here how ketogenic states are induced through a type of intermittent fast. Essentially, you fast from caloric intake and reach a state of ketosis. This is a very distinct reaction that the body is equipped with, acting as a survival instinct of the most evolved form.

Cutting back carbohydrates may seem simple but we need to realize that bread is off limits, as well as other starchy foods like rice and potatoes. A standard for ketogenic structured diets s to cut back carbohydrate consumption to 50-60 grams per day or less. Keep this up for five or six days and the body will begin to produce ketones. Now the body is forced to use stored fat for energy. This is literally shedding your excess fat. This state should not be kept up for too long or a detrimental effect can occur. Ketoacidosis can be very dangerous as the blood becomes too acidic. This is not a desired result of ketogenic diets. Be wise when practicing this diet and always listen to your body.

So the Ketogenic diet is probably the most effective to achieve healthy weight loss but should be reserved for those who have experience with intermittent fasting and other dieting experiences.

Chapter 11: Recipes

Breakfast

Zucchini Omelette

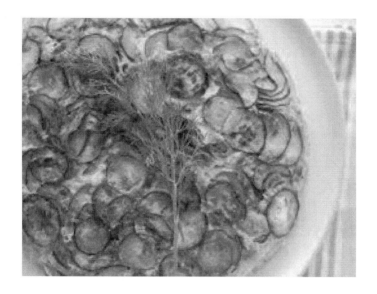

Servings: 6

Preparation time: 4 minutes

Cooking time: 3 hours and 30 minutes

Ingredients:

- 1½ cups red onion, chopped
- 1 tablespoon olive oil

- 2 garlic cloves, minced
- 2 teaspoons fresh basil, chopped
- 6 eggs, whisked
- A pinch of sea salt and black pepper
- 8 cups zucchini, sliced
- 6 ounces fresh tomatoes, peeled, crushed

Instructions:

1. In a bowl, mix all the ingredients except the oil and the basil.
2. Grease the slow cooker with the oil, spread the omelette mix in the bowl, cover and cook on low for 3 hours and 30 minutes.
3. Divide the omelette between plates, sprinkle the basil on top and serve for breakfast.

Chili Omelette

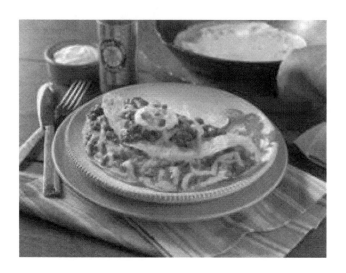

Servings: 4

Preparation time: 5 minutes

Cooking time: 3 hours and 30 minutes

Ingredients:

- 2 garlic cloves, minced
- 1 tablespoon olive oil
- 1 red bell pepper, chopped
- 1 small yellow onion, chopped
- 1 teaspoon chili powder
- 2 tablespoons tomato puree
- ½ teaspoon sweet paprika
- A pinch of salt and black pepper

- 1 tablespoon parsley, chopped
- 4 eggs, whisked

Instructions:

1. In a bowl, mix all the ingredients except the oil and the parsley and whisk them well.
2. Grease the slow cooker with the oil, add the egg mixture, cover and cook on low for 3 hours and 30 minutes.
3. Divide the omelette between plates, sprinkle the parsley on top and serve for breakfast.

Basil and Cherry Tomato Breakfast

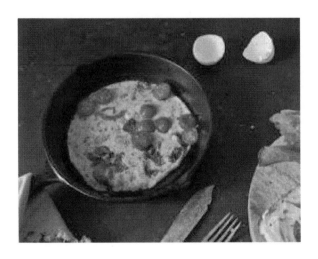

Servings: 4

Cooking time: 4 hours

Preparation time: 4 minutes

Ingredients:

- 1 tablespoon olive oil
- 2 yellow onions, chopped
- 2 pounds cherry tomatoes, halved
- 3 tablespoons tomato puree
- 2 garlic cloves, minced
- A pinch of sea salt and black pepper
- 1 bunch basil, chopped

Instructions:

1. Grease the slow cooker with the oil, add all the ingredients, cover and cook on high for 4 hours.
2. Stir the mixture, divide it into bowls and serve for breakfast.

Carrot Breakfast Salad

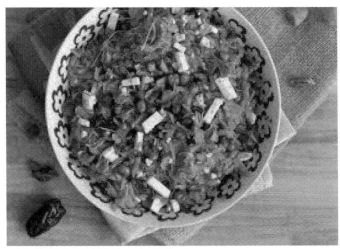

Servings: 4

Preparation time: 5 minutes

Cooking time: 4 hours

Ingredients:

- 2 tablespoons olive oil
- 2 pounds baby carrots, peeled and halved
- 3 garlic cloves, minced
- 2 yellow onions, chopped
- ½ cup vegetable stock
- 1/3 cup tomatoes, crushed
- A pinch of salt and black pepper

Instructions:

1. In your slow cooker, combine all the ingredients, cover and cook on high for 4 hours.
2. Divide into bowls and serve for breakfast.

Garlic Zucchini Mix

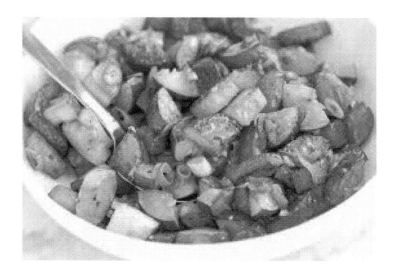

Servings: 6

Preparation time: 5 minutes

Cooking time: 6 hours

Ingredients:

-   4 cups zucchinis, sliced
-   2 tablespoons olive oil

- 1 teaspoon Italian seasoning
- A pinch of salt and black pepper
- 1 teaspoon garlic powder

Instructions:

1. In your slow cooker, mix all the ingredients, cover and cook on Low for 6 hours.
2. Divide into bowls and serve for breakfast.

Crustless Broccoli Sun-dried Tomato Quiche

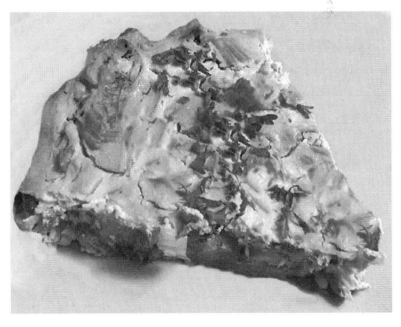

Servings: 6

Preparation time: 4 minutes

Cooking time: 3 hours and 30 minutes

Ingredients:

- 12.3-ounce box extra-firm tofu drained and dried
- 1 ½ cup broccoli, chopped
- 2 leeks, cleaned and sliced; both white and green parts
- 2 tablespoons vegetable broth
- 3 tablespoons nutritional yeast
- 2 chopped cloves of garlic
- 1 lemon, juiced
- 2 teaspoons yellow mustard
- 1 tablespoon tahini
- 1 tablespoon cornstarch
- ¼ cup old fashioned oats
- ½ teaspoon turmeric
- 3-4 dashes Tabasco sauce
- ½-1 teaspoon salt
- ½ cup artichoke hearts, chopped
- 2/3 cup tomatoes, sun-dried, soaked in hot water
- 1/8 cup vegetable broth

Instructions:

1. Preheat your oven to 375° F.
2. Prepare a 9" pie plate or springform pan with parchment paper or cooking spray.

3. Put all of the leeks and broccoli on a cookie sheet and drizzle with vegetable broth, salt, and pepper. Bake for about 20-30 min.

4. In the meantime, add the tofu, garlic, nutritional yeast, lemon juice, mustard, tahini, cornstarch, oats, turmeric, salt, and a few dashes of Tabasco in a food processor. When the mixture is smooth, taste for heat and add more Tabasco as needed.

5. Place cooked vegetables with artichoke hearts and tomatoes in a large bowl. With a spatula, scrape in tofu mixture from the processor. Mix carefully, so all of the vegetables are well distributed. If the mixture seems too dry, add a little vegetable broth or water.

6. Add mixture to pie plate muffin tins, or springform pan and spread evenly.

7. Bake for about 35 min. or until lightly browned.

8. Cool before serving. It is delicious, both warm and chilled!

Chocolate Pancakes

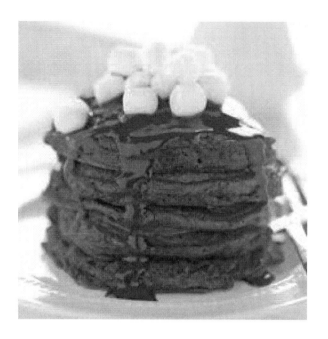

Servings: 6

Preparation time: 5 minutes

Cooking time: 80 minutes

Ingredients:

- 1 ¼ cup gluten-free flour of choice
- 1 tablespoon ground flaxseed
- 1 tablespoon baking powder
- 3 tablespoons nutritional yeast
- 2 tablespoons unsweetened cocoa powder
- ¼ teaspoon of sea salt

- 1 cup unsweetened, unflavored almond milk

- 1 tablespoon vegan mini chocolate chips (optional)

- 1 teaspoon vanilla extract

- ¼ teaspoon stevia powder or 1 tablespoon pure maple syrup

- 1 tablespoon apple cider vinegar

- ¼ cup unsweetened applesauce.

Instructions:

1. Get a medium bowl and mix all the dry ingredients (flour, baking powder, flaxseed, cocoa powder, yeast, salt, and optional chocolate chips). Whisk until evenly combined.

2. In a separate small bowl, combine wet ingredients except for the applesauce (almond milk, vanilla extract, apple cider vinegar, maple syrup, or stevia powder).

3. Add wet ingredient mixture and applesauce to the dry ingredients and mix by hand until ingredients are just combined.

4. The batter should sit for 10 minutes. It will rise and thicken, possibly doubling in size.

5. Heat an electric griddle or nonstick skillet to medium heat and spray with a small amount of nonstick spray, if desired. Scoop batter into 3-inch rounds. Much like traditional pancakes, bubbles will start to appear. When bubbles start to burst, flip pancakes and cook for 1-2 minutes. Yields 12 pancakes.

Breakfast Scramble

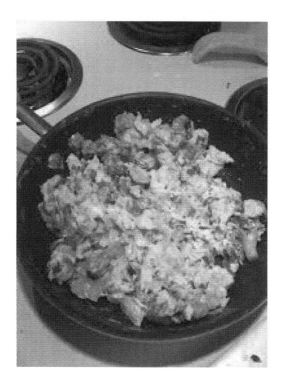

Servings: 7

Preparation time: 5 minutes

Cooking time: 60 minutes

Ingredients:

- 1 large head cauliflower, cut up
- 1 seeded, diced green bell pepper
- 1 seeded, diced red bell pepper
- 2 cups sliced mushrooms (approximately 8 oz whole mushrooms)

118

- 1 peeled, diced red onion

- 3 peeled, minced cloves of garlic

- Sea salt

- 1 ½ teaspoons turmeric

- 1–2 tablespoons of low-sodium soy sauce

- ¼ cup nutritional yeast (optional)

- ½ teaspoon black pepper

Instructions:

1. Sauté green and red peppers, mushrooms, and onion in a medium saucepan or skillet over medium-high heat until onion is translucent (should be 7–8 min). Add an occasional tablespoon or two of water to the pan to prevent vegetables from sticking.

2. Add cauliflower and cook until florets are tenders. It should be 5 to 6 minutes.

3. Add, pepper, garlic, soy sauce, turmeric, and yeast (if using) to the pan and cook for about 5 minutes.

Lunch

Vegan Tuna Salad

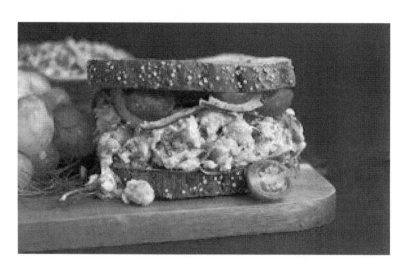

Servings: 6

Preparation time: 5 minutes

Cooking time: 55 minutes

Ingredients:

- 2 cans chickpeas
- 1 tablespoon prepared yellow mustard
- 2 tablespoons vegan mayonnaise
- 1 tablespoon jarred capers
- 2 tablespoons pickle relish

120

- ½ cup chopped celery

Instructions:

1. In a medium bowl, combine chickpeas, mustard, vegan mayo, and mustard. Pulse in a food processor or mash with a potato masher until the mixture is partially smooth with some chunks.

2. Add the remaining ingredients to the chickpea mixture and mix until combined.

3. Serve immediately or refrigerate until ready to serve.

Veggie Wrap with Apples and Spicy Hummus

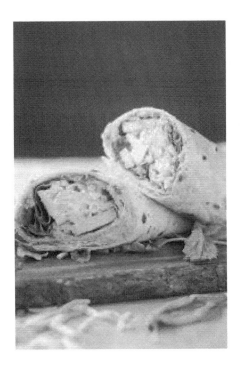

Servings: 6

Preparation time: 5 minutes

Cooking time: 40 minutes

Ingredients:

- 1 tortilla of your choice: flour, corn, gluten-free, *etc.*
- 3-4 tablespoons of your favorite spicy hummus (a plain hummus mixed with salsa is good, too!)
- A few leaves of your favorite leafy greens
- ¼ apple sliced thin
- ½ cup broccoli slaw (store-bought or homemade are both good)
- ½ teaspoon lemon juice
- 2 teaspoons dairy-free, plain, unsweetened yogurt
- Salt and pepper to taste

Instructions:

1. Mix broccoli slaw with lemon juice and yogurt. Add pepper and salt to taste and mix well.

2. Lay tortilla flat.

3. Spread hummus all over the tortilla.

4. Lay down leafy greens on hummus.

5. On one half, pile broccoli slaw over lettuce. Place apples on top of the slaw.

6. Starting with the half with slaw and apples, roll tortilla tightly.

7. Cut in half if desired and enjoy!

Turmeric Rack of Lamb

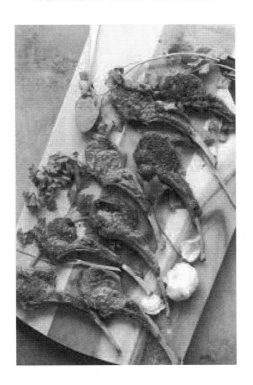

Servings: 4

Preparation time: 15 minutes

Cooking time: 16 minutes

Ingredients:

- 13 oz rack of lamb

- 1 tablespoon ground turmeric

- ½ teaspoon chili flakes

- 3 tablespoons olive oil

- 1 tablespoon balsamic vinegar

- 1 teaspoon salt

- ½ teaspoon peppercorns

- ¾ cup of water

Instructions:

1. In the shallow bowl, mix up together ground turmeric, chili flakes, olive oil, balsamic vinegar, salt, and peppercorns.
2. Brush the rack of lamb with the oily mixture generously.
3. After this, preheat grill to 380° F.
4. Place the rack of lamb in the grill and cook it for 8 minutes from each side.
5. The cooked rack of lamb should have a light crunchy crust.

Sausage Casserole

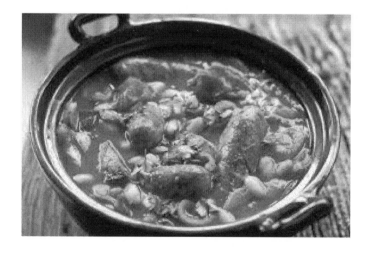

Servings: 6

Preparation time: *10 minutes*

Cooking time: 35 minutes

Ingredients:

- 2 jalapeno peppers, sliced
- 5 oz Cheddar cheese, shredded
- 9 oz sausages, chopped
- 1 tablespoon olive oil
- ½ cup spinach, chopped
- ½ cup heavy cream
- ½ teaspoon salt

Instructions:

1. Brush the casserole mold with the olive oil from inside.
2. Then put the chopped sausages in the casserole mold in one layer.
3. Add chopped spinach and sprinkle it with salt.
4. After this, add sliced jalapeno pepper.
5. Then make the layer of shredded Cheddar cheese.
6. Pour the heavy cream over the cheese.
7. Preheat the oven to 355° F.
8. Transfer the casserole in the oven and cook it for 35 minutes.
9. Use the kitchen torch to make the crunchy cheese crust of the casserole.

Cajun Pork Sliders

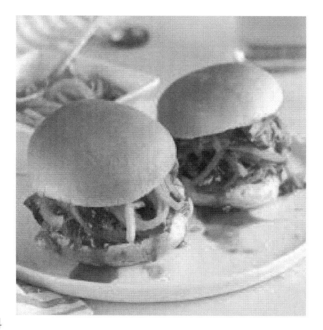

Servings: 4

Preparation time: 10 minutes

Cooking time: 45 minutes

Ingredients:

- 4 low carb bread slices
- 14 oz pork loin
- 2 tablespoons Cajun spices
- 1 tablespoon olive oil
- 1/3 cup water
- 1 teaspoon tomato sauce

Instructions:

1. Rub the pork loin with Cajun spices and place in the skillet.

2. Add olive oil and roast it over the high heat for 5 minutes from each side.

3. After this, transfer the meat in the saucepan, add tomato sauce and water.

4. Stir gently and close the lid.

5. Simmer the meat for 35 minutes.

6. Slice the cooked pork loin.

7. Place the pork sliders over the bread slices and transfer in the serving plates.

Mac and Cheese Bites

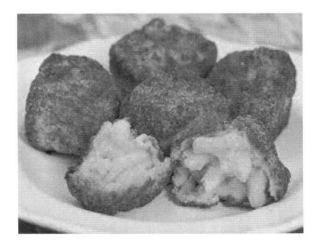

Servings: 5

Preparation time: 5 minutes

Cooking time: 50 minutes

Ingredients:

- 1 ½ cups uncooked macaroni (gluten-free will work if needed)
- 1 medium onion, chopped (can substitute with 1 medium yellow pepper if you don't care for onions.)
- 1 clove garlic, chopped
- 2 tablespoons cornstarch, or arrowroot powder
- 1 cup non-dairy milk
- ½ teaspoon smoked paprika (can substitute for chipotle powder)
- 1 teaspoon lemon juice or apple cider vinegar
- ½ cup nutritional yeast
- 1 teaspoon salt

Instructions:

1. Preheat your oven to 350° F.

2. Prepare the muffin tin with liners.

3. Prepare macaroni according to instructions.

4. While macaroni is cooking, sauté garlic and onion (or substitute of choice) until it is just starting to turn golden brown. This can be done in a dry pan, but adding some oil will work as well.

5. Add garlic, onion, and all other non-macaroni ingredients into a blender and mix until smooth.

6. Drain the macaroni and return to the pan.

7. Pour sauce over macaroni and stir well.

8. Spoon mixture into muffin tin, stirring occasionally in between such an equal amount of sauce goes in each cup.

9. Push down tops with the back of a spoon.

10. Bake in the oven for 30 min.

11. Serve once cooled.

Chicken Salad with Cranberries and Pistachios

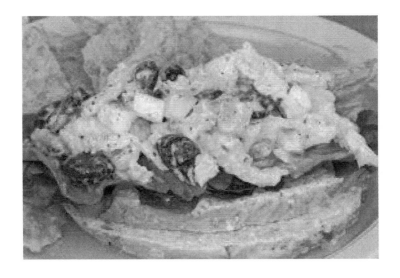

Servings: 6

Preparation time: 5 minutes

Cooking time: 80 minutes

Ingredients:

- 1 ½ cups dry soy curls (textured vegetable protein)
- 2 dashes apple cider vinegar
- ½ cup diced granny smith apples (approx. 1 small apple)
- ¼ cup shelled pistachios, chopped
- ½ cup dried cranberries
- 5-6 tablespoons veganaise (adjust depending on how creamy you would like the salad to be)
- 1 teaspoon of sea salt
- A pinch of thyme

Instructions:

1. Soak soy curls in warm water for 10 min. Squeeze excess water out of them and roughly chop larger pieces. Set aside.

2. While soy curls are soaking, mix diced apple and vinegar. Drain any excess liquid.

3. Combine apples with all other ingredients in large bowl until ingredients are evenly mixed. Add seasoning to taste. Chill for at least 30 minutes. Serve as desired.

Dinner

Pan-fried Jackfruit over Pasta with Lemon Coconut Cream Sauce

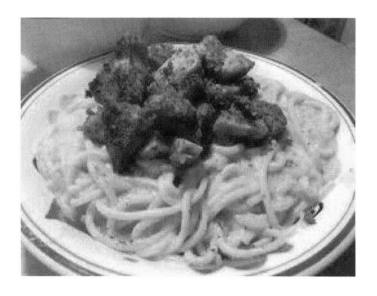

Servings: 6

Preparation time: 5 minutes

Cooking time: 30 minutes

Ingredients:

- 1 lb. pasta of choice
- 2 cans jackfruit in brine
- 2 tablespoons flour of choice
- Garlic powder, dried oregano, paprika, black pepper, kosher salt to taste

- 2 tablespoons vegetable oil

- 4 tablespoons vegan butter

- 2 cups of coconut milk

- Juice of 1 lemon

- 2 tablespoons grated vegan parmesan cheese

- 1 pinch ground nutmeg

- 1 teaspoon lemon zest (can use the same lemon from juice)

- Fresh basil leaves, chopped for garnish

Instructions:

1. Cook pasta until al dente. Drain the pasta but reserve 1 cup of the pasta water. Set it aside for now.

2. While the pasta is cooking, drain the jackfruit and cut each piece in half. Pat jackfruit dry.

3. Mix flour with garlic powder, oregano, paprika, pepper, and salt in a separate bowl.

4. Toss flour mixture with jackfruit.

5. Heat vegetable oil in a skillet. Pan-fry the jackfruit until crisp on both sides. It takes around ten minutes in total.

6. Transfer the jackfruit to a plate lined with a paper towel and set aside.

7. In a large saucepan or skillet, melt vegan butter. Add coconut milk and lemon juice. Then add parmesan cheese and nutmeg. Cook until sauce is thick.

8. Add cooked pasta and half of the reserved pasta water to skillet. Toss to coat all pasta.

9. Cook until everything is hot and the sauce is to desired consistency and pasta is heated through. If the sauce is too thick, continue to use remaining pasta water.

10. Turn off heat. Add lemon zest and add pepper and salt to taste. Sprinkle parmesan and basil leaves. Add pan-fried jackfruit on top when serving.

Butternut Squash Tacos with Tempeh Chorizo

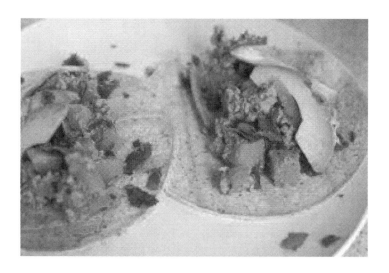

Servings: 5

Preparation time: 5 minutes

Cooking time: 50 minutes

134

Ingredients:

- One 8-ounce package tempeh
- ½ cup of filtered water
- ¼ cup apple cider vinegar
- 2 cups butternut squash, peeled, cut into cubes
- 1 teaspoon chili powder
- ½ teaspoon smoked paprika
- ½ teaspoon cumin
- ½ teaspoon garlic powder
- ½ teaspoon oregano
- A dash of cayenne
- 1 tablespoon nutritional yeast
- A few dashes of liquid smoke
- Black pepper and sea salt to taste
- ½ cup thinly julienned carrot (optional)
- 8 corn tortillas (or whatever you have on hand)
- 1 large avocado, pitted and sliced
- Cilantro, chopped

Instructions:

1. Cut the tempeh into two parts. Steam for 10 min. Place in a large bowl and tear apart into small pieces either with your hands (after it's cooled) or with a pastry cutter.

2. While tempeh is steaming, bring water and vinegar to a boil in a small skillet.

3. Add spices, squash, liquid smoke, nutritional yeast, and a pinch of sea salt to skillet. Coat well and simmer covered, stirring occasionally. Add carrots and tempeh, covering again. Simmer a little while longer, stirring to prevent sticking. Uncover and season with pepper and salt.

4. Fill warmed tortillas with squash and tempeh mix and top with avocado and cilantro.

Coated Cauliflower Head

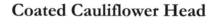

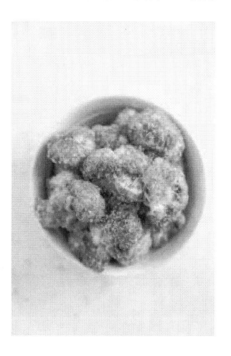

Servings: 6

Preparation time: 10 minutes

Cooking time: 40 minutes

Ingredients:

- 2-pound cauliflower head
- 3 tablespoons olive oil
- 1 tablespoon butter, softened
- 1 teaspoon ground coriander
- 1 teaspoon salt
- 1 egg, whisked
- 1 teaspoon dried cilantro
- 1 teaspoon dried oregano
- 1 teaspoon tahini paste

Instructions:

1. Trim cauliflower head if needed.
2. Preheat oven to 350° F.
3. In the mixing bowl, mix up together olive oil, softened butter, ground coriander, salt, whisked egg, dried cilantro, dried oregano, and tahini paste.
4. Then brush the cauliflower head with this mixture generously and transfer in the tray.
5. Bake the cauliflower head for 40 minutes.
6. Brush it with the remaining oil mixture every 10 minutes.

Artichoke Petals Bites

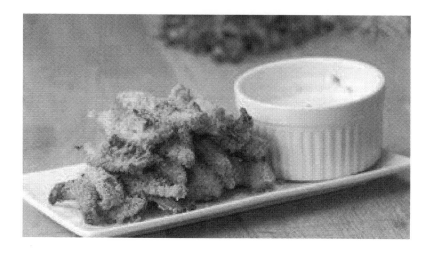

Servings: 8

Preparation time: 10 minutes

Cooking time: 10 minutes

Ingredients:

- 8 oz artichoke petals, boiled, drained, without salt
- ½ cup almond flour
- 4 oz Parmesan, grated
- 2 tablespoons almond butter, melted

Instructions:

1. In the mixing bowl, mix up together almond flour and grated Parmesan.
2. Preheat the oven to 355° F.

3. Dip the artichoke petals in the almond butter and then coat in the almond flour mixture.

4. Place them in the tray.

5. Transfer the tray in the preheated oven and cook the petals for 10 minutes.

6. Chill the cooked petal bites little before serving.

Stuffed Beef Loin in Sticky Sauce

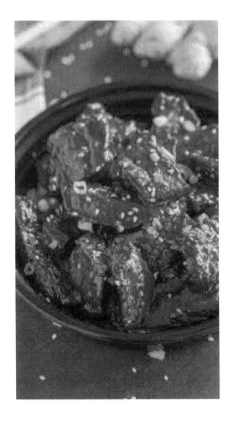

Servings: 4

Preparation time: 15 minutes

Cooking time: 6 minutes

Ingredients:

- 1 tablespoon Erythritol
- 1 tablespoon lemon juice
- 4 tablespoons water
- 1 tablespoon butter
- ½ teaspoon tomato sauce
- ¼ teaspoon dried rosemary
- 9 oz beef loin
- 3 oz celery root, grated
- 3 oz bacon, sliced
- 1 tablespoon walnuts, chopped
- ¾ teaspoon garlic, diced
- 2 teaspoons butter
- 1 tablespoon olive oil
- 1 teaspoon salt
- ½ cup of water

Instructions:

1. Cut the beef loin into the layer and spread it with the dried rosemary, butter, and salt.
2. Then place over the beef loin: grated celery root, sliced bacon, walnuts, and diced garlic.
3. Roll the beef loin and brush it with olive oil.
4. Secure the meat with the help of the toothpicks.

5. Place it in the tray and add a ½ cup of water.

6. Cook the meat in the preheated to 365° F oven for 40 minutes.

7. Meanwhile, make the sticky sauce: mix up together Erythritol, lemon juice, 4 tablespoons of water, and butter.

8. Preheat the mixture until it starts to boil.

9. Then add tomato sauce and whisk it well.

10. Bring the sauce to boil and remove from the heat.

11. When the beef loin is cooked, remove it from the oven and brush with the cooked sticky sauce very generously.

12. Slice the beef roll and sprinkle with the remaining sauce.

Vegan Fish Sticks and Tartar Sauce

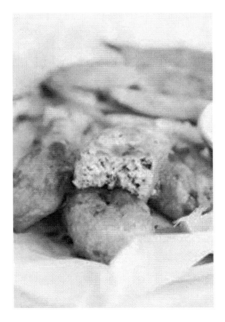

Servings: 6

Preparation time: 5 minutes

Cooking time: 80 minutes

Ingredients:

- *Fish Sticks:*

- 12-ounce package extra-firm tofu
- ½ cup cornmeal
- 1 tablespoon garlic powder
- 1 tablespoon dried basil
- 2 tablespoons dulse flakes
- 1 tablespoon onion powder
- ½ cup whole wheat flour (rice flour is a good gluten-free option)
- 10 turns fresh black pepper
- 1 tablespoon of sea salt
- ¼ cup non-dairy milk, unsweetened
- 1 cup high-heat oil for frying

- *Vegan Tartar Sauce:*
- ¼ cup sweet pickle relish
- ½ cup vegan mayo
- ½ teaspoon sugar
- ½ teaspoon lemon juice
- 5 turns fresh black pepper

Instructions:

1. Rinse tofu and drain in a colander. Placing a heavy plate on tofu with a heavy item on top will help drain better. Set it aside.

2. In a medium bowl, mix the flour, cornmeal, garlic powder, basil, onion powder, dulse flakes, pepper, and salt. Whisk together. Set the mix aside.

3. Set tofu on cutting board. Cut into quarters.

4. Slice tofu into thin pieces. You should have 28-32 pieces in total.

5. In a large cast-iron skillet, heat oil on medium/low heat.

6. In a small bowl, pour non-dairy milk.

7. Dip each piece of tofu in non-dairy milk. Immediately dip in breading, coating all sides evenly. Repeat until all pieces are coated.

8. The oil will start to splatter when hot enough. At that point, add tofu pieces to skillet. Repeat until all pieces are cooked.

9. Each side will cook for about 2-3 minutes. Watch for golden brown color. Place tofu pieces on a brown paper bag as you remove them from pan to soak up excess oil.

10. Repeat as necessary until all tofu is cooked. Cool before serving. Mix all tartar sauce ingredients until an even and creamy sauce is made. Enjoy!

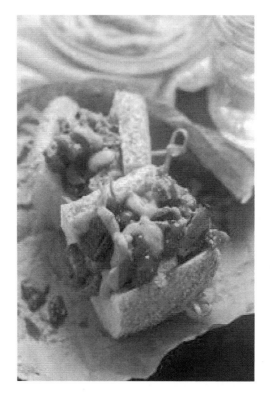

Vegan Philly Cheesesteak

Servings: 4

Preparation time: 5 minutes

Cooking time: 40 minutes

Ingredients:

- 6-8 sliced Portobello mushrooms

144

- 4 cloves garlic, minced

- 1 tablespoon olive oil

- 1 whole clove garlic

- ½ teaspoon black pepper

- 1 teaspoon dried thyme

- ½ large diced onion

- A dash of kosher salt

- 1 tablespoon vegan Worcestershire sauce

- Hoagie rolls or another small loaf of bread of choice

- 1 cup shredded vegan cheddar cheese

- Vegan mayo (optional)

Instructions:

1. Preheat the broiler.

2. In a deep skillet, heat olive oil. Brown mushrooms in oil, about 10 min.

3. Add thyme, garlic, and pepper until evenly coated.

4. Add onion and salt. Mushrooms must be well cooked before adding salt. Cook until onion is caramelized and softened, which should be for about 5 minutes. Add Worcestershire sauce and mix well.

5. Slice the bread lengthwise. Coat open sides of bread with olive oil or cooking spray. To add garlic flavor, cut the whole garlic clove, cut off the tip, and put on the oiled side of bread. Garlic powder is also a good substitute.

6. If desired, add optional vegan mayo. Place bread on cookie sheet. Fill loaves with mushrooms and top with shredded vegan cheddar cheese.

7. Place in broiler until cheese has melted, which should be 4-5 minutes.

Desserts

Mango Lime Chia Pudding

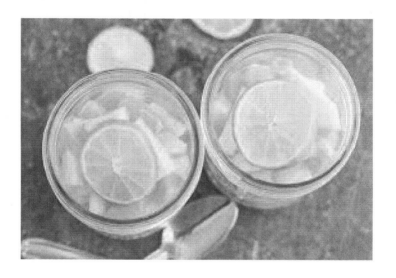

Servings: 3

Preparation time: 5 minutes

Cooking time: 30 minutes

Ingredients:

- 3 cups fresh or frozen mango chunks
- One 15.5-ounce can coconut milk
- 1 tablespoon lime zest

- ¼ cup maple syrup
- ¼ cup freshly squeezed lime juice
- ¼ cup hemp seeds
- 1/3 cup chia seeds
- *Topping options:* Approximately 8 cups of any combination of mango, banana, pineapple, or any fruit you'd love with mango and lime. (Banana is a fruit you'd want to wait to add until you are ready to eat the pudding as it browns and gets mushy very quickly once out of its peel)

Instructions:

1. Place mango chunks, coconut milk, lime zest, and maple syrup in a blender. Mix until smooth.

2. Add hemp and chia seeds in the blender and stir by hand or blend on low to just combine.

3. This should yield 4 cups of pudding. Portion it as you prefer. One suggestion is to divide into 8 portions, one each in a pint jar, and top with one cup of fresh fruit.

4. Refrigerate pudding until ready to eat, minimum 4 hours to set. The pudding keeps for 5-7 days.

Mint Chocolate Truffle Larabar Bites

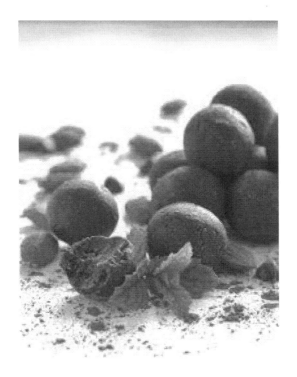

Servings: 6

Preparation time: 5 minutes

Cooking time: 45 minutes

Ingredients:

- 1 cup vegan chocolate chips (semi-sweet dark chips are recommended)
- 10 large Medjool dates
- 1 ½ cups of raw almonds
- ¼ cup coconut flour

- ¼ cup of cocoa powder
- ¼-1/2 teaspoon peppermint extract
- 2 tablespoons water

Instructions:

1. Pour almonds into a food processor and chop until a fine flour.

2. Add chocolate chips, dates, flour and cocoa, and process again until well combined.

3. Add oil and peppermint extract.

4. Process one more time until the mix starts balling up.

5. Taste a small bit and add more peppermint if you wish. Process again if you do.

6. Remove the blade from the processor and form the dough into balls. Choose whatever size you like, as they do not need to bake and will be good in any portion.

Keto Chocolate Mousse

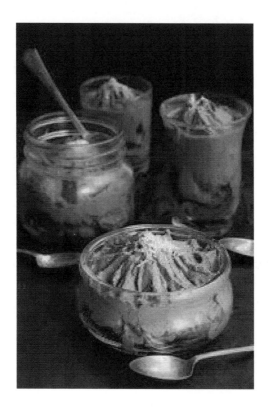

Servings: 6

Preparation time: 5 minutes

Cooking time: 40 minutes

Ingredients:

- Cocoa powder – .33 cup
- Lakanto monk fruit sweetener – 2 tablespoons
- Heavy whipping cream – 1.5 cups

Instructions:

1. Place the heavy cream in a bowl and use a hand mixer or stand mixer to beat it on medium speed.

2. Once the cream begins to thicken, add the monk fruit sweetener and cocoa and continue to beat it until stiff peaks form.

3. Serve the mousse immediately or store it in the fridge for up to twenty-four hours before enjoying it. If desired, you can serve it with Lily's stevia-sweetened chocolate for chunks.

No-Bake Peanut Butter Pie

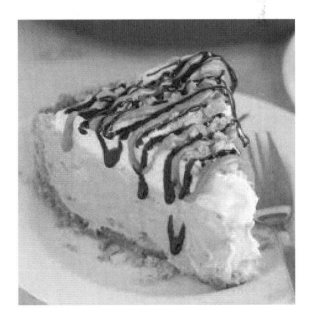

Servings: 6

Preparation time: 5 minutes

Cooking time: 60 minutes

Ingredients:

- Almond flour – 1 cup
- Butter softened – 2 tablespoons
- Vanilla - .5 teaspoon
- Lakanto monk fruit sweetener – 1.5 tablespoons
- Cocoa powder – 3 tablespoons
- Cream cheese softened – 16 ounces
- Heavy cream – .75 cup
- Vanilla – 2 teaspoons
- Swerve confectioner's sweetener - .66 cup
- Peanut butter or Sun Butter, unsweetened – .75 cup

Instructions:

1. Combine the almond flour, butter, .5 teaspoon of vanilla, Lakanto sweetener, and cocoa powder in a bowl with a fork until it forms a crumbly mixture. Press this mixture into a nine-inch pie plate and then allow it to chill in the fridge while you prepare the filling.

2. In a large bowl, beat together the cream cheese, peanut butter, confectioners Swerve, and remaining vanilla until light and creamy. Using a spatula scrape down the sides of the bowl before adding in the heavy cream.

3. Beat the filling some more until the heavy cream is incorporated and the mixture is once again light and creamy.

4. Pour the filling into the prepared crust and allow it to chill for two hours before serving. Slice and enjoy.

Strawberries with Ricotta Cream

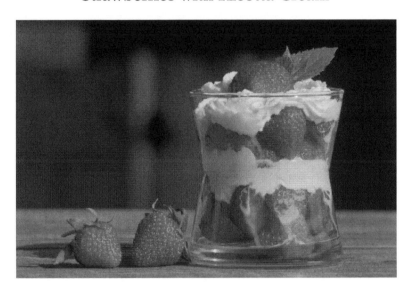

Servings: 6

Preparation time: 5 minutes

Cooking time: 40 minutes

Ingredients:

- Ricotta, whole milk – 1.5 cups

- Heavy cream – 2 tablespoons

- Lemon zest – 1.5 teaspoons

- Swerve confectioner's sweetener – .25 cup

- Vanilla extract – 1 teaspoon

- Blackberries - .5 cup

- Raspberries - .5 cup
- Blueberries - .5 cup

Instructions:

1. In a large bowl, add all of the ingredients, except for the berries, and whip them together with a hand mixer until completely smooth.

2. Set out four parfait glasses and divide half of the berries between all of them. Top the berries with half of the ricotta mixture, the remaining half of the berries, and lastly, the second half of the ricotta mixture.

3. Serve the parfaits immediately or within the next 24 hours.

Easy Chocolate Pudding

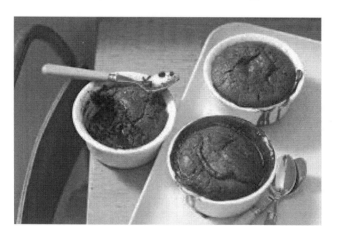

Servings: 6

Preparation time: 5 minutes

Cooking time: 30 minutes

Ingredients:

- 1 ½ cups organic coconut cream from a can
- ½ cup raw cacao powder (sifted unsweetened cocoa powder works as well)
- 6 tablespoons pure maple syrup (may adjust to up to 8 tablespoons, depending on how sweet you like it)
- 2 teaspoons pure vanilla extract
- Fine-grain sea salt

Instructions:

1. In a small saucepan over low heat, whisk coconut cream, cacao, and maple syrup until smooth. A smaller whisk my make a smoother mixture. Continue to cook over low/medium for 2 minutes, or until the mixture just starts to come to a boil with small bubbles.

2. Remove from heat. Add salt and vanilla. Stir. Taste and add more maple if you'd like a sweeter pudding.

3. Pour into individual containers/bowls or keep in one larger bowl to set.

4. Cover and refrigerate until set, or overnight for a thick and creamy pudding. Make 4 servings.

Chapter 12: 7 Day Meal Plan

DAY	BREAKFAST	LUNCH	DINNER	DESSERT
1.	Zucchini Omelet	Vegan Tuna Salad	Pan-fried Jackfruit over Pasta with Lemon Coconut Cream Sauce	Mango Lime Chia Pudding
2.	Chili Omelet	Veggie Wrap with Apples and Spicy Hummus	Butternut Squash Tacos with Tempeh Chorizo	Mint Chocolate Truffle Larabar Bites
3.	Basil and Cherry Tomato Breakfast	Turmeric Rack of Lamb	Coated Cauliflower Head	Keto Chocolate Mousse
4.	Carrot Breakfast Salad	Sausage Casserole	Artichoke Petals Bites	No-Bake Peanut Butter Pie
5.	Garlic Zucchini Mix	Cajun Pork Sliders	Stuffed Beef Loin in Sticky Sauce	Berries with Ricotta Cream

6.	Crustless Broccoli Sun-dried Tomato Quiche	Mac and Cheese Bites	Vegan Fish Sticks and Tartar Sauce	Easy Chocolate Pudding
7.	Chocolate Pancakes	Chicken Salad with Cranberries and Pistachios	Vegan Philly Cheesesteak	Mango Lime Chia Pudding

Conclusion

Intermittent fasting is an amazing concept not only for losing weight but also for gaining holistic health benefits.

It is free of cost and easy to follow. This book was an attempt to explain the concept of intermittent fasting and the ways in which it can be incorporated in daily life for best results. This book is especially for women as there are some differences in intermittent fasting methods for men and women. This book caters to the concept of intermittent fasting for women.

It explains the reasons for the difficult weight loss journey experienced by women and the ways in which it can be made easier and productive.

If you've been postponing your fast, now is the best time to start. Getting healthy is a matter of life and death, quite literally. Do not let procrastination cost you your health, and possibly your life. Some of the people dealing with lifestyle diseases today wish they had taken such a move earlier.

Get an accountability partner to walk with you, or find a community of intermittent fasting enthusiasts. If you can't find them in your area, you can do so online. With a supportive company, you'll have an easier time getting into the fast and staying on course.

Keep your expectations realistic; especially on weight loss. Results vary from one individual to the other, so don't worry too much when you can't seem to lose as much weight as the others on the same plan. With persistence and disciple, you will begin to experience the positive changes pretty soon. Go on and enjoy your leaner body, improved body image, active lifestyle and a life free from the worries of disease. The truth is: your healthy diet is not entirely about what you eat. It is also about when you eat! By eating in a way that follows your body's natural rhythms and needs, you maximize its ability to function healthily. This supports your body with everything from weight loss and muscle gain to balancing hormones and blood sugar levels. There are many different benefits that you stand to gain when you monitor not only what you eat, but when.

Perhaps one of the best parts of intermittent fasting is that this unique diet does not require you to give up on anything that you truly enjoy eating. Instead, you simply change when you eat and enjoy less healthy food choices in moderation. Of course, if you prefer to combine intermittent fasting with another diet, such as the ketogenic diet, then you will have adjusted food requirements. However, the intermittent fasting diet itself does not require you to adjust your food intake to meet any specific needs.

It is also important that you take the time to regularly monitor your symptoms and pay attention to your needs. Listen to your body and what it is telling you, as this will support you in really embracing the diet in the most powerful way possible. You do not want to find yourself struggling to succeed because you have made it too challenging for yourself. Going slower and learning to truly listen to your needs now will make your long-term goals far more achievable and sustainable.

Thank you, and best of luck!

ANTI-INFLAMMATORY DIET

THE ULTIMATE GUIDE TO HEAL THE IMMUNE SYSTEM, REDUCE INFLAMMATION AND WEIGHT LOSS WITH EASY AND HEALTHY RECIPES

By Susan Lombardi

Table of Contents

Introduction

The anti-inflammatory diet aims at ridding the body of toxins and chemicals in most normal diets and giving the body the building blocks, and it needs to heal. Reduction of inflammation can help prevent serious health problems, including heart disease and autoimmune disorders. Research suggests that the inflammation parts an important role in many of the chronic health problems which are growing in age. The anti-inflammatory diet is full of naturally occurring, whole, healthy foods. Perhaps the most important component of an anti-inflammatory diet is fruits and vegetables. Since plant-based foods are a natural source of essential vitamins and minerals, they can provide the nutrients we need without all the calories. The best vegetables are dark leafy greens like kale or spinach, which are rich in nutrients and contain antioxidants and anti-inflammatory compounds.

For a sweet treat, eat a handful of antioxidant-rich berries, or some potassium-rich banana. Don't have to be boring on salads; with carrots, peas, onions, and more to top your greens. Dairy is not banned from an anti-inflammatory diet, but experts recommend reducing the amount of whole-fat dairy that we eat when inflammation is an issue. Dairy contains plenty of saturated fat, which may increase the risk of cholesterol and heart disease, and this may reverse the champions ' good diet. Some cheeses, like feta, are, of course, better for you than their refined counterparts and can avoid the need to completely eliminate milk. Alternatives to butter, like olive oil, can also help to reduce intake.

The anti-inflammatory diet is not only a low-carbs diet, and therefore the addition of whole-grain bread, whole-grain pasta, brown rice, and other grains into meals is allowed. However, it is best to eat only whole grains, and avoid foods made from white flour and high in sugar. One excellent source is oatmeal, such as quinoa, brown rice, and many others. These whole-grain foods contain lots of fiber, promoting healthy digestion and reducing inflammation on the whole body. Use these to make salads, grain bowls, and healthy side dishes. Seafood is an important complement to an anti-inflammatory diet. If you don't like salmon, that is a popular choice, choose a milder fish like tilapia, trout or arctic char. Many fish have high omega-3 fatty acid levels that help fight inflammation and promote heart health. At least try eating seafood twice a week, preferably rather than red meat, particularly processed meat.

In volatile conditions, the book thoroughly discussed all these food components and their functions.

Chapter 1: Inflammation

Inflammation is a crucial part of the immune system's reaction to injury and infection. It is the way the body activates the immune system for healing and restoring damaged tissue, and it protects itself against foreign invaders, such as viruses and bacteria. Wounds would fester as a physiological response without treatment, and infections may turn deadly. It can, however, become problematic if the inflammatory process goes on for a longer period of time or if the inflammatory process occurs in places where it is not necessary. Chronic inflammation has been related to certain diseases such as heart disease or stroke, and can also lead to disorders that are autoimmune such as rheumatoid arthritis and lupus. But a healthy diet and lifestyle will help keep the inflammation under control.

1.1. What is Inflammation?

Consider inflammation as the body's natural response in defending itself against damage. There are two types: acute and chronic. You are probably more familiar with the acute form that happens when you strike your knee or cut your finger. Your immune system dispatches an army of WBCs that surround and protect the body, causing noticeable redness and swelling. If you contract an illness such as flu or pneumonia, the process works similarly. In these conditions, however, inflammation is necessary— without it, injuries could become festering, and simple infections could be life-threatening.

But chronic inflammation can also present in response to other unhealthy substances in the body, such as toxins from cigarette smoke or an excess of fat cells (especially belly fat). Inflammation within the arteries helps kick off atherosclerosis— the formation of a plaque that is high in fat and cholesterol. The body considers this plaque as strange and alien, so it tries to wall away from the plaque from the blood that flows in. But if that wall splits, then the plaque breaks. The contents then combine with blood, forming a clot that blocks blood flow. These clots are responsible for the bulk of heart attacks and most strokes.

A simple blood test, known as the hsCRP test, can measure C-reactive protein (CRP), which is an inflammatory marker for artery inflammation. Harvard researchers found almost 20 years ago that men with higher CRP levels— around 2 milligrams per liter (mg / L) or higher — have three times the risk of heart attack and half the risk of stroke as that in men with low or no chronic inflammation. Researchers also found that the most beneficial to people with the highest degree of arterial inflammation was aspirin, a drug that helps prevent blood clots and also dampens inflammation.

Yet several doctors do not routinely recommend the hsCRP test, because they do not feel the results will primarily impact the condition. If you're young and healthy, and you're at low risk for heart disease, there's no proof that knowing your CRP level is beneficial. If you have cardiac disease, you should already take medicines such as a cholesterol-lowering statin, which reduces the risk of heart attacks. Statins do appear to work especially well, as with aspirin, in people with arterial inflammation. One research has also found that statins decrease the risk of death in individuals with normal cholesterol levels but CRP levels of 2 mg / L or greater. So, if you are middle-aged or over and have signs of potential heart problems, such as high blood pressure level, high cholesterol level, or a family history of heart disease, knowing that you have a high level of CRP that leads you into more proactive heart safety actions. These include regular aerobic exercise, and weight loss (if necessary), and avoidance of smoking.

1.2. Types of Inflammation

There are two types of inflammation:
- Acute inflammation
- Chronic Inflammation

Acute Inflammation

Acute inflammation accompanies a knee injury, a sprained ankle, or a sore throat. It's a short-term solution with localized effects, meaning it operates at the exact location where there is a problem. As per the National Library of Medicine, the telltale signs of acute inflammation include redness, swelling, heat, and at times pain and loss of function. Blood vessels dilate in the case of acute inflammation, blood flow increases, and white blood cells surround the injured area to promote healing, Dr. Scott Walker, a family practice physician at Gunnison Valley Hospital in Utah, said. This reaction is what makes the injured area red and gets swollen.

During the process of acute inflammation, the compromised tissue releases chemicals known as cytokines. The cytokines serve as "emergency signals" that carry immune cells, hormones, and nutrients into your body to fix the issue, Walker said.

In addition, hormone-like substances known as prostaglandins produce blood clots to regenerate damaged tissue and, as part of the healing process, cause pain and fever too. The acute inflammation slowly subsides as the body heals.

Chronic Inflammation

Like acute inflammation, chronic inflammation can have long-term and whole-body consequences. Chronic inflammation is also called chronic, low-grade inflammation because it causes a constant, low-level inflammation throughout the body, as measured by a small rise in immune system markers found in blood or tissue. This form of systemic inflammation can contribute to the development of the disease, according to a review in the Johns Hopkins Health Review.

Low levels of inflammation can be caused by a perceived internal threat, even when there isn't a disease to combat or an injury to treat, and sometimes this gives signals to the immune system to answer. Because of this, white blood cells swarm but have nothing to do and nowhere to go, and they may eventually start targeting internal organs or other healthy tissues and cells, Walker said.

Scientists are researching to understand the effects of chronic inflammation on the body and the processes involved in the procedure, but it's famous for playing a role in the development of a lot of diseases.

For example, heart disease and stroke have been related to chronic inflammation. One theory suggests that when inflammatory cells stay in blood vessels for too long, they promote plaque formation. According to the (AHA), the body finds this plaque to be a foreign agent that does not belong, so it seeks to wall off the plaque from the blood flowing within the arteries. When the plaque is unstable and ruptures, it forms a clot blocking the flow of blood to the heart and brain, causing a heart attack or stroke.

Cancer is another chronic inflammation-related illness. According to the National Cancer Institute, chronic inflammation can cause damage to the DNA over time and contribute to some forms of cancer.

Chronic, low-grade inflammation often does not have signs, but doctors will check for C-reactive protein (CRP), a proxy for inflammation in the blood. High levels of CRP have been associated with an increased risk of heart disease. CRP levels can also signify an illness, or a chronic inflammatory condition, such as rheumatoid arthritis or lupus, according to the Mayo Clinic.

In addition to finding clues in the blood, a person's diet, lifestyle habits, and exposures to the environment may lead to chronic inflammation. In order to keep inflammation in check, it is necessary to maintain a healthy lifestyle.

1.3. The Pathophysiology of Inflammation

There are three sub-phases in the initial phase of inflammation: acute, sub-acute, and chronic (or proliferative). The acute phase usually lasts 1–3 days and is marked by five classical signs: heat, redness, swelling, pain, and loss of function. The subacute phase can last from 3–4 days to ~ one month, and corresponds to a required pre-repair cleaning stage. If the subacute phase is not resolved within ~1 mo, then the inflammation is said to be chronic and may last several months. The tissue can degenerate, and chronic inflammation in the locomotive system can cause tearing and fracturing. While tissue can be patched and replaced after the subacute inflammatory period during the remodeling cycle.

From a mechanistic point of view, the immediate response to tissue damage occurs in the microcirculation at the injury site. Initially, arterioles are temporarily constricted; however, chemical mediators released at the site will relax arteriolar smooth muscle within a few minutes, leading to vasodilatation and increased capillary permeability. The protein-rich fluid then exudes from the capillaries into the interstitial space. This fluid includes many of the plasma components that mediate the inflammatory response, including albumin, fibrinogen, kinins, complements, and immunoglobulins.

The sub-acute cycle is characterized by moving the phagocytic cells to the site of injury. Reacting to adhesion, molecules released from activated endothelial cells, leukocytes, platelets, and erythrocytes into damaged vessels become sticky and bind to the endothelial cell surfaces. The first cells to enter the harm site, such as neutrophils, are polymorphonuclear leukocytes. Basophils and eosinophils are more common in allergic reactions or in parasites. When inflammation progresses, the macrophages predominate, selectively attacking damaged cells or tissues. If the cause of the injury is removed, then the sub-acute phase of inflammation that follows a period of tissue repair. Fibrinolysis removes the blood clots, and fibroblasts, collagen, or endothelial cells repair or replace weakened tissues. The new collagen produced during the repair phase (mainly type III) is gradually replaced by type I collagen, in order to conform to the original tissue during the remodeling process. However, if inflammation is chronic, the tissue and/or fibrosis can deteriorate further.

1.4. Chemical Mediators of Inflammation

Biochemical mediators released during inflammation amplify and spread the inflammatory response (see the Inflammatory Mediator Actions). These mediators are soluble, diffusible molecules and can act locally and systemically. Plasma-derived mediators include complimentary, and regulated peptides and kinins. Released through the classic or alternative pathways of the supplement cascade, complement-derived peptides (C3a, C3b, and C5a) enhance vascular permeability, cause smooth muscle contraction, stimulate leukocytes, and induce mast cell degranulation. C5a is an important chemical component for neutrophils and mononuclear phagocytes. The kinins are important inflammatory mediums too. Bradykinin is the most active kinin that increases vascular permeability and vasodilation and, most importantly, promotes the release of arachidonic acid (AA) by phospholipase A2 (PLA2). Bradykinin is also a big mediator involved in the pain response. Other mediators are derived from damaged tissue or leukocyte cells, which are recruited to the site of inflammation. The serotonin and histamine vasoactive amines produce mast cells, platelets, and basophilia. Histamine induces arteriolar dilation, increased capillary permeability, smooth non-vascular muscle contraction, and eosinophilic chemotaxis, and may induce nociceptors of the pain response. The release is caused by complements from C3a and C5a, and lysosomal proteins released from neutrophils. Histamine activity is regulated by activation of one of four specific histamine receptors, called H1, H2, H3, or H4, in target cells. The majority of histamine-induced vascular effects are mediated by H1 receptors. H2 receptors mediate certain vascular effects but are more important due to their role in the histamine-caused gastric secretion. The function of H3 receptors, which may be located at the CNS, is less understood. H4 receptors are present on hematopoietic cells, and H4 antagonists are promising drug candidates for treating inflammatory conditions that involve mast cells and eosinophils (allergic conditions). Serotonin (5-hydroxytryptamine) is a vasoactive, associated histamine mediator present in the GI and CNS tracts of mast cells and platelets. Serotonin also enhances vascular permeability, dilates capillaries, and causes smooth muscle contraction, which is non-vascular. In few species, including rodents and domestic ruminants, serotonin may be the dominant vasoactive amine.

Cytokines, including IL 1–10, tumor necrosis factor α (TNF-α), and interferon γ (INF-α), are generated predominantly by macrophages and lymphocytes, but can also be synthesized by other cell types. When it comes to inflammation, their function is complex. These polypeptides modulate the actions of other cells and function towards organizing and controlling the inflammatory response. Two of the most effective cytokines, interleukin-1 (IL-1) and TNF-α, mobilize and activate leucocytes, increase the proliferation of B and T cells and increase the cytotoxicity of the natural killer cells, and are involved in the biological response to endotoxins. IL-1, IL-6, and TNF-α mediate acute phase response and pyrexia that may accompany the infection and may cause

177

systemic clinical signs, including sleep and anorexia. In the acute phase response, interleukins enable the liver to synthesize acute-phase proteins, including the complement components, protease inhibitors, and metal-binding proteins. Cytokines are also necessary to induce PLA2 by increasing concentrations of intracellular Ca2+ in the leukocytes. Colony-stimulating factors are cytokines that promote the expansion of neutrophil, eosinophil, and macrophage colonies by the bone marrow. CytokinesIL-1, IL-6, and TNF-α contribute to the activation of fibroblasts and osteoblasts in chronic inflammation and the excretion of enzymes such as collagenase and stromelysin that can activate cartilage and bone resorption. Experimental evidence also confirms that cytokines stimulate synovial cells and chondrocytes to trigger the pain-causing mediators.

Inflammatory response, lipid-derived autacoids play a major role and are a major focus of research into new anti-inflammatory drugs. Such compounds include eicosanoids such as prostaglandins, prostacyclin, leukotrienes, and thromboxane A, as well as modified phospholipids such as the platelet-activating factor (PAF). Eicosanoids are synthesized from twenty-carbon polyunsaturated fatty acids by many cells, including activated leukocytes, mast cells, and platelets, and thus are widely distributed. Hormones and other inflammatory mediators (TNF-α, bradykinin) either stimulate eicosanoid production by direct PLA2 activation or indirectly by raising intracellular Ca2 + concentrations that activate the enzyme in turn. Damage to the cell membrane may also lead to increased intracellular Ca2+. Activated PLA2 immediately hydrolyzes AA, which is quickly metabolized through one of two enzyme pathways— the cyclooxygenase (COX) pathway that contributes to the formation of prostaglandin and thromboxanes, or the5-lipoxygenase (5-LOX) pathway that produces leukotrienes.

Cyclooxygenase catalyzes the oxygenation of AA in order to form the closely related cyclic endoperoxide PGG2, which is converted to PGH2. PGG2 and PGH2 are both inherently unstable and easily transformed into separate prostaglandins, prostacyclin (PGI1), and thromboxane A2 (TXA2). PGE1, PGE2, and PGI1 are active arteriolar dilators in most species ' vascular beds, which enhance the efficacy of other mediators by increasing the permeability of small veins. Other prostaglandins, which include thromboxane and PGF2α, cause smooth muscle contraction, and vasoconstriction. Prostaglandins sensitize nociceptors to pain-provoking mediators like bradykinin and histamine and can stimulate high concentrations of sensory nerve endings directly. TXA2 is a potent aggregator of platelets that participate in thrombus production.

5-LOX catalyzes the development of toxic AA hydroxy peroxides, found mainly in platelets, leukocytes, and lungs. Then, these hydroxy peroxides are converted to peptide leukotrienes. Leukotriene B4 (LTB4) and5-hydroxyeicosatetranoate (5-HETE) are strong chemoattractant that improve polymorphonuclear leucocyte movement. LTB4 also promotes the development of cytokine in neutrophils, monocytes, and eosinophils and enhances C3b receptor expression. Many leukotrienes induce the release of histamine and many autacoids from the mast cells and promote bronchiolar constriction and mucous secretion. In a few species, leukotrienes C4 and D4 are more involved in contracting the bronchial smooth muscle than histamine.

179

The platelet-activating factor (PAF) is also derived from PLA2 activity in the phospholipids in the cell membrane. Synthesized with mast cells, platelets, neutrophils, and eosinophils, PAF induces platelet aggregation and stimulates platelets for the development of vasoactive amines and thromboxane synthesis. PAF also increases vascular permeability and causes neutrophil aggregation and degranulation.

The function of the free radical gas Nitric Oxide in inflammation is well known. NO is an efficient cell signaling transmitter through a wide array of physiological and pathophysiological processes. Tiny amounts of NO play a part in maintaining the vascular tone resting, vasodilating, and anti-aggregating platelets. Reaction to certain cytokines (TNF-α, IL-1), and other inflammatory mediators promotes the production of relatively large amounts of NO. NO is a potent vasodilator in larger quantities, causes macrophage-induced cytotoxicity, and can contribute to joint damage in certain types of arthritis.

1.5. Symptoms of Inflammation

The inflammatory effects vary depending on whether the reaction is chronic or acute.

The acronym PRISH will describe the symptoms of acute inflammation. These include Pain: The inflamed area is likely to be painful, especially during and after the touch. They release chemicals that activate nerve endings and make the area more receptive.

Redness: This is because blood fills underlying capillaries more than average.

Immobility: Inflammatory area can cause some loss of function.

Swelling: That causes an accumulation of fluid.

Heat: More blood flows into the area affected, which makes the touch feel warm.

The five acute inflammatory signs apply only to inflammations in the skin. If inflammation happens deep inside the body, in an internal organ, for example, only some of the symptoms may be visible.

For example, few internal organs may not have neighboring sensory nerve endings, so no pain should occur, as in some types of lung inflammation.

Chronic inflammatory signs have a common form. These can include:

- Nausea
- Mouth sores
- Stomach pain
- Rash
- Joint pain

1.6. Causes of Inflammation

Inflammation is due to a number of physical reactions caused by the immune system in response to an infection or physical injury. Inflammation doesn't mean that there is an infection, but an infection may cause inflammation. Three key processes occur before and during acute inflammation: The small branches of the arteries expand as blood is transported to the affected area, resulting in increased blood flow.

Capillaries are safer for fluid and protein penetration, so they can travel between the cells and the blood.

Neutrophils discharged into the body. A neutrophil is a type of WBC filled with minuscule sacs that contain digestive enzymes and micro-organisms.

Chapter 2: Chronic Inflammation, Inflammatory Diseases and their Societal and Economic pressures

Inflammation is a critical response to possible signs of danger and damage to organs in our body.

For conditions such as rheumatoid arthritis, lupus, ulcerative colitis, Crohn's disease, and other illnesses, the immune system acts against the body's tissues. Such painful and, in some cases, slowly crippling conditions may put a toll on human quality of life and establish social and economic burdens.

Within the body, the inflammatory process plays an important function in preventing and repairing injury. It may take two basic forms, acute and chronic, commonly referred to as a cascade of inflammation, or simply an inflammation. The body's immediate response to injury or attack due to physical trauma, illness, stress, or all three combinations is acute inflammation, part of the immune response. Acute inflammation helps prevent additional damage and supports the healing and regeneration process.

Nonetheless, this can lead to chronic or long-term inflammation when inflammation becomes self-perpetuating. This is called chronic inflammation and will last beyond the actual injury; for months or even years at times. It can become a problem itself and requires medical intervention to manage or avoid further inflammation-induced damage.

Chronic inflammation may have an effect on any single body part. Also, inflammation can be a side component of many diseases. For example, in atherosclerosis or artery hardening where chronic blood vessel walls inflammation may lead to plaque build-up in the arteries, arterial or vascular blockages, and heart disease. Chronic inflammation also parts a significant role in many diseases and conditions; chronic pain, reduced sleep quality, obesity, physical disability, and decreased overall patient quality.

2.1. Societal and Economic pressures of Chronic Inflammation

Chronic inflammation may also serve as a stimulator for several carcinomas. Persistent inflammation is linked with DNA damage, which in turn can lead to cancer. For example, individuals with chronic inflammatory bowel diseases (IBD) that are Crohn's disease (CD) and ulcerative colitis (UC) have an increased risk of colon cancer. The evidence suggests that over the last three decades, there has been a dramatic increase in the number of people suffering from chronic disorders like cardiovascular diseases, diabetes, respiratory diseases, autoimmune diseases, and cancers. The increasing number of these illnesses suggests that chronic inflammation, caused by excessive and inappropriate inflammatory behavior, which in turn leads to chronic inflammatory activation in the body, may contribute to the pathology of these diseases. More evidence suggests that effective chronic inflammation therapy (i.e., reducing inflammation) can reduce the risk of cardiovascular disease.

While it is difficult to measure the actual economic impact of chronic inflammation since it spreads to almost all areas of chronic disease, certain common chronic inflammation-mediated diseases can be investigated. For example, Direct healthcare costs incurred in Europe by IBD-affected patients were estimated at € 4.6–5.6 billion per year.

Health inequalities in chronic inflammatory diseases are widespread; Black Americans, for example, are 3 to 4 times more likely to have chronic kidney disease-related morbidity and mortality than white Americans.

The expense of chronic obstructive pulmonary disease (COPD) in the US was estimated at about $50 billion in 2010, including $30 billion in direct health care expenditures and $20 billion in indirect spending. The combined direct and indirect costs of UK Economic Burden NHS due to COPD were calculated at £ 982 million. In Europe, the annual cost of treating COPD is estimated at € 38.6 billion.

Chronic diseases may worsen depression symptoms and even depressive disorders, leading to chronic diseases.

2.2. Rheumatoid Arthritis

Rheumatoid arthritis is a chronic inflammatory condition (possibly affecting the entire body) that usually affects the small joints in the hands and feet. RA is an inflammatory disease in which a person's immune system attacks joint tissues and probably other body parts/organs for unexplained reasons. Symptoms can spread as the disease progresses to the wrists, knees, ankles, elbows, hips, and shoulders. Consequently, RA causes the joints to suffer from discomfort, inflammation and ultimately damage and malformation. RA may cause people to feel ill, exhausted, and feverish; it also symmetrically affects joints where the pain in the joint is felt on both sides of the body.17- RA is markedly different from osteoarthritis (OA), a degenerative joint disease that only limits joint function. However, pediatric arthritis and rheumatological disorders have affected approximately 294,000 children under the age of 18 in the US. The most common age of onset among women is between 30 and 60 years, whereas it occurs later in men's lives. Per-patient costs for uninsured Rheumatoid Arthritis patients were estimated at $5,758, which is aggregated to an annual total expense of $560 million when weighted by uninsured prevalence. In the United Kingdom, the National Audit Office (NAO) found that in 2009, RA cost about £560 million per year to the National Health Service (NHS), with the majority of this spending in the acute sector, and that the total expense was calculated at around £560 million per year.

Studies show that an increase in early treatment for RA patients would bring significant productivity benefits, with economic gains of £ 31 m due to decreased sick leave and job losses. According to the NAO of the United Kingdom, 10 percent of RA patients are treated within three months of the onset of symptoms; economic analysis suggests that increasing this to 20 percent can cause cost increases, but faster treatment may become cost-neutral after nearly nine years.

2.3. Psoriatic Arthritis

Psoriatic arthritis is an inflammatory arthritis type that can sometimes be serious, a chronic, autoimmune disease. Nearly 30 per cent of chronic

187

skin psoriasis patients will also develop psoriatic arthritis. Patients with PSA inflammation will also experience painful swelling in hand and wrist joints. In addition, PSA may also develop this type of psoriatic arthritis. Many patients also experience physical disabilities due to their PSA, reduced emotional well-being and general tiredness. This in turn leads to direct medical costs from the use of health care services. The resulting functional limitations lead to indirect costs such as disability and lost productivity, and are significant drivers of total care costs. In the US, the direct annual health care costs for PSA are estimated to be as high as $1.9 billion, based on an average cost per patient of $3,638.36. A European analysis found a total direct cost of $4,008 in Hungary.

2.4. Inflammatory Bowel Disease (IBD), ulcerative colitis (UC) and Crohn's disease (CD)

Inflammatory intestinal disease (IBD) identifies disorders of chronic or persistent immune response and gastrointestinal (GI) tract inflammation. Ulcerative colitis (UC) and Crohn's disease (CD) are the two most common inflammatory bowel diseases.

UC mainly affects the large intestine, while any part of the GI tract may be affected by CD. Symptoms of UC often include blood and mucus-containing diarrhea, severe cramp-like abdominal pain, anemia, loss of appetite, weight loss, fatigue, strong bowel movement desire, and tenesmus (incomplete evacuation sensation). Individuals with moderate to severe UC reported negative effects on education, jobs, social/personal life, relationships, and depression. Surveys have shown anxiety and stress that people with UC complain about their disease.

More than seventy percent of people with UC have reported symptoms affecting their ability to enjoy leisure activities, and nearly two-thirds report their symptoms of UC influencing their work performance. About 1.6 million Americans have IBD, an increase of around 200,000 since this statistic was last recorded by the Crohn's and Colitis Foundation of America in 2011.

Up to 70,000, new cases of IBD are diagnosed annually in the United States. In the United States, there could be as many as 80,000 children with IBD.44 In 2012, there were nearly 233,000 Canadians living with IBD (129,000 persons with CD and 104,000 persons with (UC). An approximate 2,5–3 million people in Europe suffer from IBD. In Asia, we are seeing growing incidence of IBD. Thirty years ago, with IBD, Hong Kong was home to less than 1 in 1 million people. Today about 3 out of 100,000 people in Hong Kong are diagnosed with new IBDs.

2.5. Chronic obstructive pulmonary disease (COPD)

Chronic pulmonary obstructive disease (COPD) develops as an effective, chronic

Half of COPD patients face movement restrictions due to health problems compared to 17 percent of patients without COPD. Many people with COPD (38%) report having difficulty walking or climbing stairs, compared to those without the condition (11%). Many people with COPD (22 percent) claim they need to use special equipment for health problems compared with 7 percent without COPD among adults. COPD is the third-most-common cause of death in the United States. It is estimated 3 million people in the United Kingdom suffer from COPD.

And the disease kills about 30,000 people a year, more than breast, bowel, or penile cancer. France has 3.5 million COPD sufferers (6 percent adult incidence) and 16,000 deaths every year.

2.6. Treatment of Chronic Inflammation

Although acute inflammation is part of the animal body's natural system of protection against injury and disease, chronic inflammation in itself is considered a disease. Because chronic inflammation affects specific areas of the body and can be associated with a defined disease process, treatment approaches vary considerably.49 Physicians have relied on steroids for decades to suppress immune response. Steroids, though an effective choice, come with common side effects such as weight gain and potentially harmful side effects such as heart enlargement and liver cancer. Today, as science has progressed, new classes of therapies have been developed which transform inflammatory disease management by targeting other main proteins and body pathways. Today, patients with chronic inflammation and inflammatory disease have new treatment choices with more targeted agents that go beyond wide-ranging immunosuppressive therapies.

Scientists' ability to better understand the underlying biology of the disease and identify groups of patients can lead to new and innovative medicines through precision medicine, which will best respond to certain treatments.

Chapter 3: Arthritis is an Inflammatory Disease

Inflammatory arthritis is a phrase used to describe a group of conditions that affect the immune system. This means that your body's defense system starts attacking your own tissues rather than germs, viruses, and other foreign substances that can cause pain, stiffness, and joint damage. These are also known for being autoimmune diseases. Inflammatory arthritis has three most common forms: rheumatoid arthritis, ankylosing spondylitis, psoriatic arthritis. These illnesses are also called systemic diseases since they can affect the whole body. They can happen at any age.

Such diseases are still not healed, but the outlook for those afflicted with inflammatory arthritis is much better than it was 20–30 years ago. Effective treatment begins much earlier, and new drugs are available, which means less joint damage, less need for surgery, and fewer complications.

Inflammatory arthritis is not the same as osteoarthritis that happens when the cartilage inside the joint is rubbed away.

The inflammatory arthritis route is a guide to what information is available and could be of help to you at any major point of your journey, from first detected symptoms to specialist care if the disease progresses. The route guides you through each process to relevant organizations and sources of information.

Steps to Arthritic Pathway

Step 1–Recognizing symptoms prior to seeking medical help

You can experience joint and/or back pain at Step 1, but your GP has not yet looked at the symptoms. You might have seen a few of the following two posters warning individuals of one of the three most severe types of inflammatory arthritis: rheumatoid arthritis, ankylosing spondylitis, and psoriatic arthritis.

The Squeeze Test is the most common measure for rheumatoid arthritis and psoriatic arthritis that includes pushing the patient's hand or foot across the knuckle joints, as shown. If this examination is unduly painful, then there may be signs of those conditions.

Test A gives an MCP (metacarpophalangeal) test.

Test B shows an MTP (Metatarsophalangeal) test.

If you have signs that may be associated with inflammatory arthritis, don't delay and seek help from your GP as soon as possible.

Phase 2–First time visiting the doctor:

At Step 2, you'll see your doctor first. The following links will help with your first GP visit, handle your symptoms, and get general health advice. There is also some information that you might find helpful while waiting for your first specialist appointment, which should be within 4–6 weeks.

Inflammatory arthritis can, at times, be difficult to diagnose, and usually, only a rheumatologist specialist or a GP with a specific interest in musculoskeletal disorder (GPWSI) may make a firm diagnosis. Since the various causes of inflammatory arthritis are treated by specialist teams led by a rheumatologist doctor and are usually hospital-based, but not always, this is a specialized treatment area. This means that they may not have the level of experience, skill, and knowledge needed to make a clinical diagnosis unless your GP has been qualified to be a specialist in addition.

There's no one test that you can take to tell if you're getting rheumatoid arthritis, ankylosing spondylitis, or psoriatic arthritis, so it's essential that if your GP feels you're having either of those disorders, they'll refer you to a rheumatologist specialist for assessment as soon as possible.

The British Pain Society has a number of articles on pain management with in-depth advice.

The NHS Live Well pages offer general health recommendations on a variety of topics, including healthy eating, smoking cessation, and exercise.

The Patients Association has a number of manuals, including one entitled *Preparing the GP for an appointment."

Your first specialist appointment should be within four to six weeks, but it may be quicker if the waiting times in your area allow.

Phase 3–First seeing the doctor after referral:

You should see the doctor at Phase 3 (most definitely a physician for rheumatology) first. You may get a solid diagnosis during your first visit, but in the very early stages, it is sometimes difficult to diagnose inflammatory arthritis. If you have rheumatoid arthritis, ankylosing spondylitis, or psoriatic arthritis, no single test will tell you, so for diagnosis, and you may need more tests and visits.

The links below will help you with this phase in your path and will guide you to other organizations that can provide more information. It includes information about: your first medical meeting and how to make potential treatment plans for the healthcare professionals who may be interested in your treatment.

Using NICE recommendations (RA) is meant to help you understand the care and treatment facilities that should be provided in the NHS for those with rheumatoid arthritis.

We suggest you think and take note of everything you want to know before your first visit to see the expert. This will help ensure the answer to all your questions during the consultation process. It may also be helpful to have a friend or family member with you, as they may remember stuff you did not take in afterward.

Step 4–Testing, procedures and additional information

You will get your first diagnosis at Phase 4, and search for appropriate care with your specialist team. At this stage, you might need to have a number of tests to help your specialist team decide the best treatment for you. These tests could include x-ray ultrasound scans for blood test Disease activity scores. These tests may seem a bit confusing to start with, particularly when you've just been diagnosed, but your rheumatology nurse practitioner will help explain them to you on your first visit. During your first or second doctor visit, you will usually meet the rheumatology nurse practitioner. The qualified nurse will help answer a few of your possible questions.

Step 5—Continuing care in primary and specialist care:

Treatment will continue at Phase 5. You will usually see your team of specialists very often to start with, but your visits will become less regular once your team is confident that your condition is well handled.

With regular blood tests, you will need to go to your GP surgery or the hospital. These will check how you manage the disorder and how you respond to the therapy. Then, the GP will speak to the specialist team about some of the diagnosis.

You and your family will be revisiting the disease and its effects on your life at least once a year when your condition is in balance.

If you have a problem or an increase in your symptoms, it's important that you know how to get in touch. You should get access to a nurse-led helpline call.

As well as the organizations mentioned below that include person-specific information in Step 5, you may also be interested in the following general information: The Patients Association is an independent, national charity that addresses the issues and needs of patients.

The Citizens Advice Bureau offers information on health rights, which includes what assistance is available via the NHS, patient rights, health cost aid, how to make a complaint, and health care for people abroad.

Direct Government defines the assistance that may be provided across a number of topics such as education, transportation, and finance.

Most specialty teams have a line of instruction often run by the specialist nurse-making sure you know the number. Your GP is also a reliable source of aid and support.

Phase 6-Managing the long-term illness or coping with complications:

Phase 6 is an advanced disorder, affecting only a few individuals. Advanced illness may include organs such as your heart and lungs that can cause severe complications and/or other long-term conditions such as diabetes or heart disease. Other complications can rarely occur like vasculitis.

However, for those dealing with inflammatory arthritis, the situation today is significantly better than it was 20–30 years ago. Despite significant new therapies now available, and effective treatment started much earlier than it used to be, with less discomfort, less need for surgery, and fewer complications, the future is much brighter. The better you know, and how to handle your condition.

The links below give information about possible complications. You can also identify specific organizations that can assist you, including those that offer assistance to caregivers.

Chapter 4: Gastritis an Inflammatory disease – Causes, signs and symptoms, treatment and cure

Gastritis is an inflammation of a stomach lining. There are two types of acute gastritis, and a chronic one. Most people with gastritis may have no symptoms; however, both acute and chronic gastritis may have symptoms and signs of abdominal pain, diarrhea, vomiting, and sometimes belching, bloating, loss of appetite, and indigestion.

What causes an upset stomach?

A bacterium known as Helicobacter pylori and non-steroidal anti-inflammatory drugs are the major cause of gastritis, and there are many other causes of the condition too, such as infectious agents, autoimmune disorders, illnesses such as Crohn's disease, sarcoidosis, and sporadic granulomatosis gastritis. How do you know if you feel upset about your stomach?

Gastritis may be diagnosed either by examining the symptoms and history (e.g., NSAID and/or alcohol) or by testing breath, blood, urine, immunology, and biopsy for H. Pylori and other measures such as endoscopy or radiological studies show improvements in the mucosa.

4.1. Some facts about gastritis

What is Treatment for Gastritis?

Treatment with gastritis varies by source. Other less common causes may receive similar treatment, but do not address the underlying cause.

Is there a diet on gastritis?

Symptoms of gastritis can be worsened by chemical irritants, which should reduce or avoid the gastritis symptoms together. Stop smoking cigarettes, for example, reduce excessive alcohol consumption, avoid caffeinated, decaffeinated, and carbonated drinks; and fruit juices containing citric acid, such as grapefruit, peach, pineapple, etc., and avoid high-fat foods.

There is no diet for gastritis, however, and the growth of H. A diet rich in fiber and foods containing flavonoids such as certain teas, onions, garlic, berries, celery, kale, broccoli, parsley, thyme, soy products, and legumes such as lentils, kidney, green, wheat, pinto, and marine beans can prevent pylori.

Which home remedies help to ease the symptoms of gastritis?

Home remedies may help to reduce gastritis symptoms, but normally the underlying cause of the condition is not handled.

Individuals suffering from acute gastritis usually recover without complications. However, if serious complications arise, there could be a variety of results from good (early treatment) to poor for chronic gastritis. Acute gastritis complications may occur very rarely.

Chronic gastritis complications include peptic ulcer, bleeding ulcers, anemia, stomach cancers, MALT lymphoma, renal issues, tightness, intestinal inflammation, or even death.

Gastritis may also be prevented if the underlying causes of gastritis (e.g., alcohol use or use of NSAIDs) are treated or not used. Is one possible cure for gastritis?

Gastritis can be treated if it treats the cause that underlies it.

Why do you fight gastritis?

Since gastritis is an infection and can be avoided by washing your hands thoroughly and often, for example, using good hand washing techniques, avoid circumstances where you are exposed to chemical substances, radiation, or toxins in order to avoid gastritis risk.

What foods light up gastritis symptoms?

Health care professionals at Maryland University and others say eating smaller, more frequent meals and avoiding salty, acidic, fried, or fatty foods will help reduce symptoms. In fact, a reduction of stress is also advised. Dietary improvements such as ginger tea and/or honey chamomile tea allegedly relieve gastritis symptoms while H can be prevented by onions, garlic, cranberries, apples, and celery. Pylori Production.

Foods that might hamper H. Pylori growth and relief of gastritis symptoms include teas (particularly green and white) Yogurt, Peppermint, Wheat bran, Carrot juice, Coconut, water Green leafy vegetables, Onions, Garlic, Apples, Fresh fruits and berries Celery Cranberry juice, Kale, Broccoli, Scallions Parsley, Thyme, Soybeans, cSoy foods Legumes (beans, peas, and lentils). Although these home remedies can help reduce or soothe symptoms.

4.2. Causes of gastritis

Stomach mucosal infection by a bacterial species called Helicobacter pylori is a major cause of both acute as well as chronic gastritis. This bacterium usually initially acutely infects the stomach antrum (stomach mucosa without acid-producing cells) and may grow over time to infect most or all of the stomach mucosa (chronic gastritis) and remain there for years. This infection triggers an initial strong inflammatory response, and with changes in the intestinal cells, long-term chronic inflammation can eventually develop. Another main cause of acute and chronic gastritis is the use (and overuse) of non-steroidal anti-inflammatory drugs (NSAIDs).

Nevertheless, there are many other causes of gastritis; the following is a list of common causes of both acute and chronic gastritis; with repeated or persistent presence of most of these causes, chronic gastritis may occur: bacterial, viral and parasite infections.

4.3. Symptoms of gastritis

Most patients suffering from gastritis are without symptoms. The condition is only reported when other possible diseases are checked for the stomach mucosal samples. Nevertheless, as signs of gastritis develop, the most common symptoms are abdominal pain (intermittent or constant burning, squeezing or gnawing pain), nausea and vomiting, diarrhea, loss of appetite, bloating, burping, and belching.

Symptoms of gastritis come and go through time, particularly with chronic gastritis. Indigestion (dyspepsia) is also another concept that involves this cluster of symptoms. Symptoms of extreme gastritis may include prolonged diarrhea, bloody stools, and anemia.

4.4. Natural remedies for gastritis

Not all therapies would work for everyone, so a person might have to try out several of these before they find out what works best for their situation.

1. **Follow an anti-inflammatory diet:** Gastritis is also considered as inflammation of the stomach lining and eating a diet that can provide relief over time to help reduce inflammation. Nevertheless, research has not shown conclusively that gastritis is caused or avoided by eating a certain diet.

By keeping a dietary diary, people may recognize which foods cause their symptoms. We can then start to reduce their intake or avoid other foods altogether.

Foods commonly associated with inflammation are: processed foods gluten acidic foods Milky foods Spicy alcohol foods

2. Consume a garlic extract supplement: Some research suggests that garlic extract can help lower the symptoms of gastritis. Crushing and consuming raw garlic will also work well.

If a person does not like the raw taste of garlic, they might try to chop the garlic and eat it with a spoonful of peanut butter or wrapped in on a dry date. The sweet taste of the peanut butter, or date, should help mask the garlic flavor.

3. Probiotics: Probiotics can help improve digestion and facilitate regular bowel movements. Probiotic additives introduce good bacteria into a person's digestive tract that can help stop H spread.

Eating foods that contain probiotics can also improve the symptoms of gastritis. Such foods include kimchi kombucha sauerkraut kefir yogurt.

4. Drink some green, honey tea manuka. One study showed that consuming green or black tea can reduce the prevalence of H substantially, at least once a week. Gastrointestinal Pylori. Manuka honey may also be useful in that it contains antibacterial properties that help fight infection.

Many people believe warm drinking water soothes the stomach and improves digestion.

Manuka honey can be purchased online and in health-care shops.

5. Use of essential oils: Essential oils such as lemongrass and lemon verbena have been found to help improve resistance to H. Pylori in laboratory work.

Few other oils that can have a positive effect on the digestive system are peppermint, ginger, and clove.

Essential oils should not be engulfed and should always be diluted with a carrier oil when applied to the skin.

Users might want to use the oils in a diffuser or talk to a doctor about using them safely to help relieve gastritis.

It's important to remember that the AMERICAN Food and Drug Administration (FDA) does not authorize natural oils or herbal medicine.

6. Eat lighter meals: eating large, heavy carbohydrate meals can put a strain on the digestive system of a person and make gastritis worse. Eating small meals regularly during the day can help ease the digestive process and reduce the symptoms of gastritis.

7. Avoid smoking and extra use of painkillers: smoking can harm a person's stomach lining, and it also increases the chances of developing cancer in the stomach.

Taking too many pain medications over - the counter, including aspirin or ibuprofen, can also weaken the stomach lining and make gastritis even worse.

8. Reduce stress: Stress can produce gastritis flare-ups, so rising stress levels is an effective way to help manage the disease.

Strategies for stress management include Relaxation breathing exercises, sleep therapy, and yoga.

Prevention: While the cause of gastritis differs between people, certain precautions may be taken to avoid unpleasant symptoms.

Steps to reduce gastritis include: avoiding known triggering foods to stop smoking influence and reducing the stress that prevents alcohol from maintaining a healthy weight that prevents overuse-the-counter pain medications Home remedies can help many people manage gastritis. However, when symptoms do not go away, it is necessary to talk to a doctor. When to see a doctor, Patients with gastritis should see a doctor if they experience: a gastritis flare-up that lasts longer than a week, vomiting blood in the stool. A doctor may ask questions, conduct an evaluation, and may decide to perform other tests.

Common gastritis prescribed medicines include histamine blockers 2 (H2), which help to reduce the production of acid. Proton pump inhibitors (PPIs) are available in both prescription and over - the counter forms, which also work to decreases acid production and are available on the counter as well as on prescription antibiotics used to treat H. Pylori Infection.

Chapter 5: Anti-inflammatory Dietary Tips for Gastritis

Gastritis is a digestive disease that causes the stomach lining to become inflamed. Symptoms include heartburn, indigestion, diarrhea, and frequent burping. A few people will benefit from dietary changes. Gastritis has various forms and causes. Infection with Helicobacter pylori bacteria (H. pylori) is one common cause. Other causes include the use of non-steroidal anti-inflammatory drugs (NSAIDs), high intake of alcohol, and certain inflammatory disorders, such as Crohn's disease.

Some foods can add to the risk of H. Pylori infection, and certain dietary habits can cause stomach lining erosion or otherwise aggravate gastritis symptoms. A person suffering from gastritis can find eating hard, leading to loss of appetite and unwanted weight loss.

Untreated gastritis can lead to ulceration, chronic pain, and bleeding. In some cases, it can turn life-threatening. Chronic stomach inflammation also increases stomach cancer development.

5.1. Anti-inflammatory Foods to eat

No particular diet can cure gastritis, but eating certain foods can help improve or prevent the symptoms from getting worse.

Dietary changes, for example, can help protect the stomach lining and reduce inflammation.

Green tea and fresh fruits and vegetables can help to prevent gastritis in the body. They are good sources of antioxidants and can help to prevent cell damage and disease by raising the levels of reactive compounds called free radicals in the body. Aliments that may help inhibit development of H. Pylori and reduced gastritis and ulcer growth include cauliflower, swede, cabbage, radish, and other Brassica vegetable berries, such as turmeric blueberries, blackberries, raspberries, and strawberries; a mild spice that may have anti-inflammatory properties Antioxidants may also help prevent a wide range of other conditions. There you can learn more about antioxidants and the foods they include. Foods that help alleviate Gastritis symptoms include stomach lining inflammation. For this reason, an anti-inflammatory diet may be beneficial to some people.

There's no ideal anti-inflammatory diet. Eat plenty of antioxidant-rich fresh fruit, vegetables, and other plant foods to combat inflammation. It is more important to avoid processed foods and those containing unhealthy fats and to add salt or sugar.

Foods to help treat gastritis: Broccoli and yogurt are two foods that can help with gastritis care.

Broccoli contains a chemical sulforaphane which has antibacterial properties. It also includes antioxidants that can aid in the prevention of cancer. Consequently, eating broccoli sprouts can help relieve or prevent gastritis and reduce the risk of stomach cancer. An older study published in 2009 by scientists has identified participants with H. Pylori infections that ate 70 grams of broccoli sprouts per day — more than half a cup — had lower infection and inflammation levels for eight weeks than those that didn't eat broccoli.

In 2006, another team investigated whether eating around 2 cups of probiotic yogurt a day before using an antibiotic combination could improve the ability of the medication to combat drug-resistant H. Pylori. Yeah.

After four weeks, the researchers found that people who drank yogurt and antibiotics tended to kill the infection more effectively than those who just took antibiotics. The findings in the yogurt may have been obtained from the active cultures of beneficial bacteria that help improve the body's ability to fight infection.

5.2. Dietary Tips

The following dietary changes will help prevent or regulate gastritis: Eat little but often: eating five to six smaller meals throughout the day— instead of three big meals — can help reduce the accumulation of stomach acids.

Managing weight: Overweight and obesity increase the risk of developing gastritis. A doctor can help create a weight loss plan to reduce the risk of gastritis and other associated health issues.

Use antacids: A doctor may also advise on pain relief drugs.

Ask a Physician about supplements: some dietary supplements, including omega-3 fatty acids and probiotics, can reduce the effects of gastritis.

Omega-3 antioxidants and probiotic supplements can be ordered online. Still, talk to a doctor before taking these or other supplements, as they may interfere with other health issues.

Additionally, some additives, including iron, can increase the risk of gastritis. Foods that make symptoms worse include: spicy fried foods that are acidic in alcohol can sometimes cause an allergen to inflammation. In this type of case, a doctor might recommend a diet for elimination, which includes removing all food groups from the diet to see if it causes the symptoms.

One team of doctors, for example, reported that one person has a form of gastritis caused by dairy and egg. The team also had been looking at wheat, nuts, soy, fish, and rice.

Those considering an elimination diet should first speak to a physician, as it may cause nutritional deficiencies.

Foods that increase the risk of gastritis: if a person consumes: red meat processed meat products that are alcohol-pickled, fried, salted, or smoked fatty foods, Studies have shown that, for example, salty and fatty foods can affect the stomach lining. High-salt diets can change the cells within the stomach, making them more susceptible to H. Pylori.

High levels of alcohol can also cause stomach inflammation and worsen the symptoms. It can also induce an erode in the stomach lining.

Any health tips: Stop smoking to help with gastritis prevention or treatment: smoking increases the risk of inflammation, teeth, esophageal, and stomach cancer.

Reducing stress: High levels of stress can cause stomach acid to develop, which can aggravate symptoms and inflammation.

Checking any medication: Frequent use of NSAIDs may increase the risk of damage to the stomach lining, which may cause or worsen symptoms of gastritis. The aspirin, ibuprofen, and naproxen are all forms of NSAID.

5.3. Diet for stomach ulcers and gastritis

A diet of ulcer and gastritis is a meal plan that restricts foods that irritate your stomach. Most products have the ability to worsen symptoms such as stomach pain, bloating, heartburn, or indigestion.

Foods: will I limit or avoid? You might need to avoid acidic, spicy, or high-fat foods. Not every food has the same effect on everybody. You'll need to learn which foods exacerbate the symptoms and limit other foods. Some foods that could worsen the symptoms of ulcer or gastritis are as follows: beverages, whole milk, chocolate milk, Hot cocoa, and cola. Some drinks with caffeine Regular and decaffeinated coffee Peppermint and spearmint tea Green and black tea, with or without caffeine Orange and grapefruit juices. Eat whole grains, nuts, vegetables, and dairy products that are free of fat or low in fat, includes bread of whole wheat, cereals, noodles, and brown rice—select lean meats, poultry, fish, beans, nuts, and vegetables. A healthy meal plan includes low unhealthy fat levels, salt, and added sugar.

Healthy fats come from canola and olive oil. Consult a healthy meal plan with your dietitian for more.

What could further guidance help?

Do not feed only prior to bedtime. Arrange for feeding at least 2 hours prior to bedtime.

Eat small and daily meals. Small, regular meals can be more accommodating to your stomach than big meals.

Procedure AGREEMENT: You have the right to help with the planning of the procedure. To decide what care you want to get, speak with your doctor about treatment options. Yours is also the right to deny medication. The above knowledge is a pure educational aid. Talk to your GP, nurse, or pharmacist before taking any medical treatment to see if it's safe and effective for you.

Chapter 6: Obesity and Inflammation are interrelated

Obesity is a health issue that has reached widespread proportions with growing global prevalence. The global obesity epidemic increases the risk of chronic metabolic disorders. It is, therefore, an economic problem that increased the costs of the related comorbidities. Moreover, obesity has been shown to be associated with chronic systemic inflammation in recent years, and this status is caused by innate activation of the immune system in adipose tissue, which promotes increased production and release of pro-inflammatory cytokines that lead to the systemic acute-phase response characterized by elevation of acute cytokines. Therefore, a growing body of evidence confirms the important role played by the inflammatory response in obesity condition and the related pathogenesis of chronic diseases.

6.1. Obesity and Chronic Inflammation

Inflammation is a physiological response needed to restore homeostasis, which is altered by various stimuli; however, inflammation or excessive response that is permanently established may have deleterious effects. In overweight and obesity, low-grade chronic inflammation exists; recent studies have identified some of the intracellular inflammation pathways associated with these conditions; experiments in mice and humans show that the ingestion of nutrients acutely activates inflammatory responses; thus, it is believed that the starting signal of inflammation is overfeeding and that the pathway originates In ob. These kinases control downstream transcriptional programs by inducing regulation of the expression of the inflammatory mediator gene through transcription factors protein-1 activator, nuclear factor πB, and interferon regulator. The increase in cytokines exacerbates the activation of receptors by creating a positive inflammatory feedback loop and signaling the inhibitory metabolic pathways.

Inflammasomal and Toll-like receptors (TLRs) likewise activate the innate immune system. Strong evidence now suggests that inflammatory signaling plays a prominent role in developing a chronic inflammatory disorder that impairs insulin responsiveness.

6.2. The Inflammasome

The inflammasome is a sensor of the innate macromolecular immune cells which activate the inflammatory response. Recognition of various noxious signals by the inflammasome results in the activation of caspase-1, which then induces the secretion of potent proinflammatory cytokines, in particular interleukin-1β (IL-1β). In this way, inflammasome-mediated processes are important for the regulation of metabolic processes.

The inflammasome is a heptamer assembled from monomers containing Nod-like receptors (NLRs), the ASC adapter protein (an apoptosis-associated speck-like protein containing a caspase-recruitment domain), and the caspase-1 enzyme. NLRs are distinguished by a structure composed of a central realm that mediates nucleotide-binding and oligomerization and a variable N terminal area essential for protein-protein interactions. The NLR activates caspase-1, which, when assembled as an inflammasome, converts pro-IL-1β into active IL-1β.

The NLR family is made up of 22 members for humans, divided into four subfamilies, NLRA, NLRB, NLRC, and NLRP, based on their N-terminal domain configuration. We interact with the inflammasome-related proteins ASC and caspase-1. Metabolic tension, insulin resistance, and type 2 diabetes have been associated with an NLRP member named NLRP3. Inflammatory activation of NLRP3 in obesity induces macrophage-mediated activation of T cells in adipose tissue and impairs insulin sensitivity establishing a persistent pro-inflammatory condition that impairs the sensitivity of insulins. Among other substances, hyperglycemia, reactive oxygen species, palmitate, lipopolysaccharides, and uric acid can cause inflammasome activation.

Recent studies have shown that a glucose-upregulated protein, the protein that interacts with thioredoxin (TXNIP), interacts with NLRP3, resulting in IL-1β secretion and pancreatic β-cell function impairment.

6.3. The Inflammatory Cytokines and Obesity

The cause of the inflammation during obesity and the underlying molecular mechanisms causing its prevalence are not fully understood, but pro-inflammatory cytokines play a central role. In obesity, inflammatory cytokines show higher circulating concentrations than in lean beings, and they are believed to play a role in insulin resistance induction. The adipose tissue is the primary source of pro-inflammatory cytokines in obesity; it is released primarily through macrophage

214

infiltration, while adipocytes play a role. Thus, the blood levels of these cytokines are reduced after weight loss. The main cytokines responsible for chronic inflammation are the tumor necrosis factor-αy, interleukin-6, and the inflammasome-activated IL-1β.

TNF-α is a pleiotropic molecule that parts a central role in inflammation, immune system production, apoptosis, and lipid metabolism, having numerous effects in adipose tissue, including lipid metabolism and insulin signaling—circulating TNF-α increases in obesity and declines in weight loss. TNF-α stimulates IL-6 release, another strong pro-inflammatory cytokine, and reduces anti-inflammatory cytokines such as adiponectin. TNF-α induces adipocyte apoptosis and encourages insulin resistance by inhibiting a signaling pathway for the insulin receptor substratum.

It is a cytokine that plays significant roles in the development of acute phase reactions, inflammation, hematopoiesis, metabolism of the bone, and cancer. It controls energy homeostasis and inflammation; it may inhibit the production of lipoprotein lipase, and influences hypothalamic appetite and energy intake is important for the transition from acute to chronic inflammatory disease. For conditions such as obesity, insulin resistance, inflammatory intestinal disease, inflammatory arthritis, and sepsis, this leads to chronic inflammation when deregulated.

IL-1β is a pyrogenic cytokine. It is primarily developed by blood monocytes as a response to infection, injury, or immunological threat; this causes fever, hypotension, and the production of additional pro-inflammatory cytokines such as IL-6. IL-1β is formed from its pro-IL-1β inactive counterpart by an inflammasome. But IL-1β has now emerged as a leading instigator of the pro-inflammatory response to obesity. Significant progress has been made in the last decade in understanding the role of cytokines and the inflammasome in obesity, chronic inflammation, and type 2 diabetes. Also, further work is needed to better understand the underlying mechanisms, since they are possible points of intervention in the quest for new therapeutic modalities for these global health problems.

6.4. Markers of Inflammation in Obesity

Many chronic diseases include an inflammatory response marked by a rise in cytokines and serum concentrations of acute-phase reactants such as fibrinogen, C-reactive protein (CRP), complement, serum amyloid A, haptoglobin, sialic acid and low concentrations of albumin. Acute-phase reactants are made in the liver, and cytokines, includingIL-6 and TNF-alpha, regulate its production. Considered the classic sensitive acute-phase reactant, the CRP is a very sensitive systemic inflammation marker, and its serum concentration is rapidly increasing as a response to a variety of stimuli. Under normal conditions, this protein is found in low concentrations.

Visceral adipose tissue can generate inflammatory mediators that cause acute-phase reactants to be generated in hepatocytes and endothelial cells. Perhaps because adipocytes have been shown to express and secrete TNF-alpha, adipose body mass may be an important mediator in understanding the relationship between obesity and inflammation. Several studies have shown that abdominal adiposity is correlated with CRP level elevation, independent of the body mass index (BMI), which is a general adiposity scale. In those individuals with abdominal adiposity, the proportion of people with elevated hs-CRP was significantly higher than control subjects, although they had a comparable BMI. This is a pro-inflammatory cytokine synthesized with adipose, endothelial, macrophage, and lymphocyte tissue. In the liver, the CRP is mainly synthesized in response to IL-6 stimuli. Obese people are at increased risk for multiple chronic diseases, of which several are often distinguished by high concentrations of CRP. Because adipose tissue is the main component of pro-inflammatory cytokines such as IL-6and TNF-alpha, both cytokines increase lipogenesis in the hepatic and cause a systemic acute-phase response.

In recent years, obesity has been shown to be associated with low-grade inflammatory processes characterized by elevated circulating levels of pro-inflammatory cytokines in healthy obese subjects such as IL-6, TNF-alpha, and acute-phase proteins (CRP and haptoglobin). This pattern is also seen in obese children who have higher levels of CRP than children with average weights. Some studies have indicated that dietary weight loss is associated with decreased circulating levels of IL-6, TNF-alpha, CRP, and other inflammation markers regardless of age, sex, and BMI. Likewise, the weight reduction observed after gastric bypass in subjects indicates a decrease in rates of CRP andIL-6.

6.5. Metabolic Syndrome

The metabolic syndrome has three or more of the following characteristics: obesity, hyperglycemia, hypertension, low HDL cholesterol levels, and/or hypertriglyceridemia. While pathogenic mechanisms are poorly understood, a central role has been assigned to the pro-inflammatory cytokine's TNF-alpha and IL-6, as both are synthesized by adipose tissue. Inflammatory activity factors such as CRP, IL-6, serum amyloid A and soluble adhesion molecules have been associated with this condition.

Risk factors: Low-grade chronic inflammation is consistent with metabolic syndrome, and some features of insulin resistance. Several studies have shown a substantial association of CRP levels with symptoms of metabolic syndrome, including adiposity, hyperinsulinemia, resistance to insulin, hypertriglyceridemia, and low cholesterol HDL. In just a few studies, the relationship between CRP and the development of metabolic syndrome has been established. In addition, elevated levels of hs-CRP have been shown to be associated with having metabolic syndrome with increased risk of adverse cardiovascular events in individuals. Inflammation was proposed as a common part of various metabolic disturbances of insulin, glucose, and lipids affecting the underlying development of the metabolic syndrome.

It has also shown that CRP has independent prognostic information on the extent of metabolic syndrome. It has been suggested that CRP is an additional component of metabolic syndrome. In one research, it was explained that elevated CRP levels (almost 3 mg / L) might increase the risk of metabolic syndrome caused by factors of obesity and resistance to insulin.

Healing counseling: Observational studies have shown that dietary patterns close to the Mediterranean diet, rich in fruits and vegetables, and high in monounsaturated fiber and fats, have resulted in reduced prevalence of metabolic syndromes. Furthermore, interventional studies have also shown a decrease in inflammatory factors following Mediterranean diets and/or national dietary guidelines in subjects with metabolic syndrome.

Work to assess inflammation pathways in individuals with metabolic syndrome is scarce; however, some have reported anti-inflammatory effects from statin therapy. Since subjects with metabolic syndrome show increased inflammation, statins may be a therapeutic alternative following improvement in the lifestyle of therapy.

6.6. Chronic Inflammation and Metabolic Syndrome

The rising incidence of obesity and metabolic syndrome is worrying. The activation of inflammatory pathways, typically used as a defense for the host, causes the severity of this illness. Inflammation activation is most likely more than one cause. Evidently, metabolic overload evokes stress responses, such as oxidative, inflammatory, organelle, and cell hypertrophy, leading to vicious cycles. For physical reasons, adipocyte hypertrophy causes cell separation and will cause an inflammatory reaction. The inability to grow adipose tissue to absorb incoming fat leads to deposition in other organs with effects on insulin resistance, especially in the liver. The oxidative stress that accompanies eating may contribute to the inflammation that is associated with obesity, particularly when fat and/or other macronutrients are overly ingested without the concomitant ingestion of antioxidant-rich foods/beverages. Furthermore, work on the interaction of microbiota with food and obesity brought with its new hypothesis for the relationship between obesity / fat diet and inflammation. Some causes, such as shifts in the psychological and/or circadian rhythms, may also result in oxidative/inflammatory status beyond these. The challenge of treating obesity / metabolic syndrome is due to its multifactorial existence, where environmental, genetic, and psychosocial causes interact through complex networks.

Metabolic syndrome prevalence increases and is high. Metabolic syndrome suggests a group of disorders including glucose intolerance, central obesity, dyslipidemia (hypertriglyceridemia, elevated no esterified fatty acids (NEFAs), and decreased cholesterol, high-density lipoprotein (HDL), and hypertension. It may manifest in several ways, depending on the combination of the various components of the disorder, and it is well known that it increases the risk of developing cardiovascular disease, type 2 diabetes, and cancer. However, how it begins and how it causally connects the different components between them is still not clear. Different groups of research paid particular attention to one aspect or another. For example, the American Association of Endocrinology does not consider obesity as a factor and emphasizes the importance of the syndrome's insulin resistance. Nevertheless, obesity and the metabolic syndrome do not completely overlap, and now there is clear evidence that there is "benign" obesity. The concentrations of adiponectin plasma in this metabolically healthy obese phenotype are high, in good agreement with the effect of adiponectin overexpression in ob. / ob. mice are resulting in the expansion of fat mass and defense against metabolic comorbidities. The original definition of the World Health

Organization considered insulin resistance to be a central feature of metabolic syndrome, whereas the more recent National Cholesterol Education Program (NECP) description: Adult Treatment Panel III (ATP III) applies equal weight to any aspect of the syndrome: glucose sensitivity, obesity, hypertension, and dyslipidemia.

Welsh et al. used a bidirectional Mendelian randomization method to investigate the causal nature of the relationship between adiposity and inflammation and concluded that higher levels of adiposity from fat mass and obesity-associated gene and melanocortin receptor 4 single nucleotide polymorphisms resulted in higher levels of C-reactive protein (CRP), with no proof of reverse trends. While this interesting finding needs to be validated and applied to other inflammatory markers, it helps in the chronic inflammation associated with metabolic syndrome that we focus on adipose tissue. Whatever their roots, whether the key initiator is obese or not, the chronic low-grade inflammatory disorder that accompanies the metabolic syndrome has been implicated in both the development of the syndrome and its related pathophysiological effects as a major player. In good agreement with this understanding of events, weight loss in obese patients is regularly tested to correlate with a reduction in inflammation biomarkers accompanied by an increase in metabolic parameters, that is, insulin sensitivity.

6.7. Cardiovascular Disease

Throughout recent years, common inflammation markers (such as CRP, IL-6, and TNF-alpha) have been identified in the prediction of coronary events; in this regard, CRP is the most important marker for cardiovascular disease.

Danger factors: Circulating high levels of inflammatory markers such as CRP, TNF-alpha, and IL-6 is associated with increased risk of developing cardiovascular disease; even certain acute-phase reactants may also lead to pathogenesis. Even though the recurrent elevation of CRP levels is in a mild degree, it is an independent predictor of future cardiovascular events even within a normal value range. Stratified CRP levels of < 1, 1– 3 and > 3 mg / L result in low, moderate and high risk of future cardiovascular events. Previous to this, multiple studies have found a significant correlation between CRP and cardiovascular risk. This finding was first observed over 50 years ago, where heightened CRP level after myocardial infarction was identified as a predictor of poor prognoses. Later, the European Concerted Research on Thrombosis and Disorders Angina Pectoris Study Group indicated that CRP concentrations were higher in patients with coronary events than in those without such events. The Cholesterol and Repeated Events Trial also showed that elevated CRP levels are associated with a significant risk of coronary events following myocardial infarction. Inflammation has been gradually becoming a strong indicator of potential cardiovascular events.

Additionally, hs-CRP is a better proxy for cardiovascular disease than other acute-phase reactants, cytokines, and molecules of soluble adhesion. Therefore, backed by a large number of observational studies and meta-analysis, CRP is considered a mediator of cardiovascular disease, regardless of age, smoking, rates of cholesterol, blood pressure, and diabetes, among other standard risk factors assessed in the clinical setup. Therefore, CRP is one of the most well-documented risk factors for the onset of cardiovascular disease care. Some interventional research using the Mediterranean diet and others marked by increased consumption of mustard or soya oil, fruits, vegetables, nuts, and whole grains decreased cardiovascular disease levels with important anti-inflammatory effects. Several observational and interventional work has shown that intakes of omega-3 and omega-6 fatty acids and alpha-linolenic acid contribute to lower cardiovascular disease incidence and lower inflammatory marker concentrations. Moreover, multiple studies have shown that statin therapy is associated with reduced inflammation and decreased risk of cardiovascular disease.

6.8. Diabetes

Researches have shown that subclinical systemic inflammation predicts diabetes development, as measured by elevated levels of CRP and IL-6[142–149]. It can actually interfere with insulin signaling by inducing proteins that bind to the insulin receptor. A growing body of evidence in this regard supports the hypothesis that chronic systemic inflammation in peripheral tissues contributes to a decrease in insulin sensitivity.

Risk factors: Several studies on healthy subjects have confirmed the relationship between insulin resistance and elevated levels of CRP and cytokines IL-6 and TNF-alpha. Moreover, it has been shown that low-grade chronic inflammation in individuals with impaired glucose tolerance is related to glucose metabolic disturbances.

223

It has been documented that TNF-alpha is overexpressed in the adipose and muscle tissues of obese and insulin-resistant nondiabetic subjects, an overexpression positively associated with insulin resistance. Ironically, the circulating TNF-alpha levels in type 2 diabetes are higher than in IFG / IGT. In addition, several cross-sectional studies demonstrated an improvement in CRP levels in patients with diabetes, and an increase in CRP, IL-6, and TNF-alpha in IGT subjects.

In addition, certain kinases such as protein kinase C isoforms, I kappa B Kinase-β, and c-jun-terminal kinase have been elevated in obesity, and these kinases have been involved in altering insulin signaling by promoting serine phosphorylation of insulin receptor substrates along with suppression of this substratum's tyrosine phosphorylation. Additionally, various studies have shown that excess nutrient and obesity are associated with elevated levels of free fatty acids that can cause both peripheral tissue insulin resistance and innate immunity activation.

Furthermore, cut-point values for determining the risk of developing the disease are difficult to set, as intermediate CRP values are at moderate risk for metabolic disturbances. Nonetheless, patients with diabetes and CRP values > 3 mg / L were reported to have a 51 % higher risk of all-cause mortality and a 44 % higher risk of cardiovascular mortality relative to those with diabetes and CRP <3 mg / L of comparable age and sex, regardless of classical risk factors such as lipids, blood pressure, and glycemia.

Healing therapy: In the clinical area, there are numerous therapeutic choices, such as genetic, biochemical, and pharmacological targeting of inflammatory signaling pathways enhancing insulin action, which is a central problem in type 2 pathophysiology of diabetes. Existing evidence for inhibiting the cascade of multiple inflammatory kinases in animal models enhances the action of insulin. Thiazolidinediones pharmacological therapies demonstrated anti-inflammatory effects that inhibited both the role of adipocytes and macrophages in obesity and type 2 diabetes. Numerous clinical studies have shown improvements in beta-cell function, and response to insulin decreases in glucose levels, the use of anti-inflammatory drugs to treat type 2 diabetes, and even pre-diabetes. In addition, other studies in patients with type 2 diabetes taking statins have shown a beneficial and additive effect on inflammation levels, which could be an alternative therapy for this condition; however, recommendations for clinical practice should be discussed about the proper use of statin therapy, as specific studies have documented contradictory results with respect to the disease.

The cause of inflammation during obesity and the underlying molecular mechanisms causing its prevalence are not yet fully understood, but pro-inflammatory cytokines do play a central role. In obesity, inflammatory cytokines show higher circulating concentrations than in lean beings, and they are suspected of playing a role in insulin resistance induction. Adipose tissue in obesity is the main source of pro-inflammatory cytokines; it is released mainly by the infiltration of macrophages, while adipocytes play a role. Obesity stems from a number of risk factors,

225

including increased energy consumption and insufficient exercise. Patients with obesity, such as cardiovascular disease, diabetes, metabolic syndrome, and NAFLD, have many difficulties predicting, among others, the risk of future cardiovascular events and death. Different mechanisms have been suggested, including antioxidant, anti-inflammatory, fiber intake, and antiestrogenic processes, to clarify the protective role of certain dietary components, in particular Mediterranean dietary components, which could be a significant change in the clinical lifestyle to prevent the development of metabolic diseases.

6.9. Athletes and Inflammation and the role of antioxidants

The endurance athletes and coaches also pose these questions: How do we preserve good health and improve performance? Are there dietary strategies that promote good health during periods of intense exercise and competitive planning? Are diet or antioxidant supplement intakes effective, and if so, which approach is best? Scientists and clinicians are also interested in these issues, and a concerted effort has been made to identify the clinical and performance effects of supplementation and the physiological mechanisms underlying it in laboratory and field-based research.

This study explores some of the important aspects of the antioxidant supplementation of endurance athletes, including increased free radical production and subsequent oxidative stress caused by high loads of endurance training, the effect of endurance training and oxidative stress on immune function, the influence of improved antioxidant status on performance, recovery and adaptation factors, two special factors.

6.10. Oxidative Stress and Endurance Training

Endurance athletes like those who participate in individual running, cycling, swimming, and triathlon events undergo multiple hours of aerobic exercise training each week. Endurance training focuses on the use of oxygen in the skeletal muscle in order to provide the energy needed for such activities. This training's oxidative nature can stimulate the production of highly reactive free radicals, and antioxidant defenses are needed to protect cells from free radical harm. This potential for destroying cells is known as oxidative stress and may result in the inflammatory response of the immune system to protect host tissues.

There is significant evidence that high-intensity or prolonged endurance-training loads promote increased free radical development and oxidative stress (Watson et al., 2005). Preparation for endurance yields increased production of reactive oxygen species (ROS) (Powers and Jackson 2008) and of reactive nitrogen species (Reid 2001; Powers and Jackson 2008). The most widely formed ROS in cells are superoxide and nitric oxide (Powers, Jackson 2008). While oxidative stress can induce an inflammatory response, free radicals can also play a significant physiological role in training adaptations. There was considerable debate about whether excessive antioxidant intake would reduce training-related adaptations (Gross et al. 2011). It may be difficult for many endurance athletes to strike the right balance between pro-oxidants and antioxidants (Atalay et al. 2006; McGinley et al. 2009).

Regular physical activity can also reduce oxidative stress and inflammation, and improve immune function (McTiernan 2008; Shanely et al. 2011). The length, intensity, and difficulty of exercise activity affects this relationship. Although high-intensity endurance training can increase the activity of antioxidant enzymes and decrease markers for exercise-induced oxidative stress (Miyazaki et al. 2001), extremely high training loads are associated with an acute reduction in antioxidant ability and an increase in oxidative stress markers (Neubauer et al. 2008). This impact has also been shown in athletes who participate in ultra-endurance events, including ultramarathons and ironman triathlons (Knez et al. 2007; Neubauer et al. 2008; Turner et al. 2011). Basically, athletes need to change exercise loads to prevent an increased risk of fatigue, illness, or injury.

Importance of antioxidants Anti-oxidants protect the body against oxidative stress and therefore prevent damage to a wide range of cellular structures, including lipids, proteins, and DNA (Martin 2008). In general, antioxidants are graded as either endogenous or exogenous in the body. The main endogenous antioxidants are superoxide dismutase, catalase, and glutathione peroxidase enzymes, and glutathione. Exogenous antioxidants come from the diet and include, but are not limited to, vitamin E (tocopherols and tocotrienols), vitamin C (ascorbic acid), coenzyme q10 and carotenoids. These compounds have different biological effects, some by converting free radicals into less reactive substances, others by binding supply-lowering proteins, and others by acting as free radical scavengers (Knez et al. 2007; Powers and Jackson 2008).

In preparation for the competition, endurance training places major acute and chronic demands on physiological, metabolic, and energetic processes. Meeting nutrient demands can be a challenge for athletes. Competition for key nutrients during prolonged exercise training between the active and immune systems is one reason that some athletes are at elevated risk of illness. Athletes, who want to add or increase their intake of antioxidants via either dietary sources or supplements, have many choices. Antioxidant supplements are increasingly being marketed in general and sporting communities, with numerous claims about enhanced energy quality, faster recovery from exercise, and improved cardiovascular and immune health. Supplement use is common among endurance athletes enrolled in college athletes in the USA with daily consumption levels of up to 90 percent (Frioland et al. 2004).

6.11. Endurance exercise and symptoms of respiratory illness

One of the most common reasons an elite athlete has to pose for medical examination (Robinson and Milne 2002) is upper respiratory symptoms, and a proven link exists between the training load and the risk of respiratory disease (Walsh et al. 2011). Many athletes suffer from recurrent upper respiratory episodes. Such symptoms are consistent with an inflammatory response and have until recently been thought to be the result of upper respiratory infection. Nonetheless, this isn't always true, and the etiology of the airway inflammation in endurance athletes is varied (Spence et al. 2007), including infection, acute inflammation, allergy, and poorly managed asthma.

While moderate amounts of exercise are usually safe, high volumes of training can increase the risk of respiratory symptoms relative to inactive or moderately active individuals (Nieman 1994). High-intensity, high-volume, or both endurance training events that trigger temporary changes in immune cell function, may be responsible for a period of increased vulnerability to infection that is clinically significant. The risk of upper respiratory tract disease is assumed to be highest during periods of overreaching or overtraining, and around competition. A period of increased vulnerability, the so-called' window of immunosuppression' after exercise, is based on data that shows that immune disturbances can last up to 72 h after competition or a hard training session (Nieman 2007).

Acute neutrophilia and lymphopenia, a decline in natural killer cell activity and T-cell function, a decline in salivary IgA, and higher in pro-inflammatory cytokines and chemokines can be summarized as follows briefly (Nieman 2007). Some changes in the cellular and soluble elements of the immune system have been well established. For these immune responses, it is believed that catecholamines, adrenaline, blood flow, body temperature, and dehydration are among the biological regulators (Nieman 2007).

The underlying infectious cause of athletes suffering from upper respiratory symptoms is not always well established. The belief that inflammation, which is not associated with infection, plays a significant role, is well known in many clinical presentations. In a study investigating the etiology of upper respiratory symptoms in elite athletes, bacterial infections accounted for only 5 percent of the presentations (Reid et al. 2004), with other inflammatory factors responsible for 30–40 percent of upper respiratory symptoms. In support of this finding, viral etiology was identified to the general population in just 30 percent of athletes with the disease with different pathogens (Spence et al. 2007). Epstein–Barr virus reactivation has been shown to be responsible for 22 percent of athletes with chronic symptoms (Reid et al. 2004). Asthma, asthma, and untreated non-breathing diseases and autoimmune disease are some causes of upper respiratory disease in athletes (Spence et al., 2007).

As a result of severe mechanical stress on the airways, exhaustion, and exposure to agents (pollutants, irritants, allergens) able to cause airway damage, athletes may also be at increased risk for airway injury. Such effects are due in large part to the huge and common air motions associated with endurance training. Oxidative stress has been identified as a major factor in contaminant-induced bronchospasm, but only a few studies have investigated the impact of these agents on respiratory symptom-induced athletes (Chimenti et al. 2009).

The treatment with antioxidants has the potential to be a valuable dietary technique for athletes at risk of respiratory disease.

Athletes on a high-antioxidant diet, or who consume antioxidant supplements, may have improved immunity from respiratory disease

231

caused by both exercise and pollution; however, research examining such recommendations are lacking. Outside the athletic culture, antioxidants are known to play a role in altering airway inflammation. As compared to a low antioxidant diet, a general community study of asthmatic individuals examined the role of a high antioxidant diet (Wood et al. 2012). In this study, the low antioxidant diet resulted in a deterioration of two commonly used indicators of asthma intensity (percentage of forced expiratory volume predicted in one second, and percentage of forced vital capability predicted, increased concentration of the inflammatory marker C-reactive protein in serum, and decreased the time for acute asthma exacerbation compared to high antioxidant levels Given the evidence that inflammation involves a significant number of upper respiratory symptoms experienced by athletes, and a significant reduction in airway inflammation is associated with increased intake of dietary antioxidants in non-athletic subjects, a comparable protection can be given to athletes by supplementing the diet with antioxidant-rich foods. More experimental work in athletic groups is required to test this hypothesis.

6.12. Effects of Inflammation on performance, recovery, and adaptation

There is only limited evidence of the correlation of decreased sports performance with respiratory inflammation and infections. A decline for results has been associated with an episode of respiratory symptoms before international competitions for elite swimmers (Pyne et al. 2005). Endurance events such as a marathon, ironman race, or triathlon can cause muscle damage and an acute inflammatory response— though there is also a related rise in anti-inflammatory cytokines (Suzuki et al. 2006). The balance between inflammatory and anti-inflammatory effects depends on a number of factors. The increase in ROS produced in the skeletal muscle during physical activity depends on the intensity and duration of the task being performed and also on the capacity to antioxidant. Though low levels of ROS activity tend to improve (in vitro) contractility, high levels can impair function. Several studies have tried to reduce the adverse effects of exercise through the use of antioxidant-rich supplements. A drop in creatinine kinase and urinary 8-hydroxy-guanosine has been reported following pre-season supplementation with a combination of antioxidants and amino acids in college soccer players (Arent et al., 2010). Although the players showed no benefit from the results, this could mean a potential gain from recovery. Acute supplementation of trained cyclists with a pine bark extract, Pycnogenol, increased fatigue time, total oxygen consumption, and performance 4 hours before an exercise trial (Bentley et al. 2012). Another research that supports the theory of increased antioxidant potential has investigated the effect of supplementing cherry juice on maximum voluntary contractions compared to an energy-matched knee extension placebo (Bowtell et al., 2010). Cherry juice supplementation significantly improved the recovery of isometric strength following exercise as compared with the placebo. While this study is not specific to endurance athletes, the results support the idea that increased availability of antioxidants can delay fatigue time and promote muscle recovery that may improve performance (Bowtell et al., 2010). Before prolonged

233

exercise (2.5 hours of running), blueberry intake resulted in higher NK cell counts and higher anti-inflammatory cytokine concentrations relative to a control group (McAnulty et al., 2011).

Quercetin is one of the few antioxidant supplements that have been tested and shown a strong performance benefit in a number of studies; however, the trials were mostly conducted using untrained subjects. A significant rise in untrained subjects was noticed in a 12-minute treadmill test running results study (Nieman et al. 2010). In another study, the mean oxygen consumption and cycle time to exhaustion were increased after seven days of quercetin supplementation as compared to placebo (Davis et al. 2010), again in untrained subjects. It is uncertain that highly trained athletes would see that benefit.

One topic of much discussion in sports nutrition is whether the use of supplements can affect normal physiological processes. Many researchers argue that antioxidant supplementation can interfere with the cellular signaling role of ROS and thus prevent adaptations required to improve performance (Gross et al. 2011). The alternative view is that dietary supplements simply increase natural antioxidant capabilities, given the very high demands associated with endurance training and overestimate the fear of physiological interference. In order to overcome this dispute, further studies are needed.

6.13. Dietary vs. Supplement sources of antioxidants

A common problem for athletes is whether they need enough nutritional supplements or antioxidant intakes from usual dietary sources. Inconclusive evidence exists that treatment with anyone antioxidant is sufficient to prevent oxidative damage from exercise-related free radicals or to prevent exercise-related immune disorders or respiratory inflammation (Nieman 2008). There's a lack of evidence to address this question in athletes. Nevertheless, the view has arisen in people with asthma that whole foods or multi-formulation supplements containing more than one antioxidant may be more effective in enhancing antioxidant capacity (Wood et al., 2012).

A Mediterranean diet allows the general population to fend off oxidative stress. The ATTICA study, a comprehensive epidemiological review of 3000 residents of urban and rural areas surrounding Greece's Athens, identified important linkages between adherence to the Mediterranean diet and health benefits (Kontogianni et al. 2012). Higher overall antioxidant ability and lower rates of low-density oxidized lipoprotein (LDL) cholesterol have been associated with good adherence to this diet. It is believed that reducing LDL-cholesterol accounts for its protective effect on cardiovascular health. This study further proved a link between the Mediterranean diet and decreases in inflammation and coagulation markers.

While a high antioxidant diet is associated with reduced inflammation of the airways and severity measures in patients with asthma and chronic airway disease (Wood et al. 2012), there is some concern about the effectiveness and even protection of supplementation with one single high-dose antioxidant. For example, experiments in the form of α-tocopherol combined with isolated vitamin E have increased oxidative stress markers, somewhat counterintuitive, over placebo during the Triathlon World Championships (Nieman et al., 2004).

A variety of dietary antioxidant supplements including quercetin, blueberries, and even cherry juice (Nieman et al. 2007, 2010; Bowtell et al. 2010; Davis et al. 2010; McAnulty et al. 2011) demonstrated the potential for improvement in exercise outcomes. Multi-nutrient supplementation may be a safer choice compared to very high doses of individual antioxidants, or nutrients that provide improved antioxidant protection, with lower potential harm risks (Atalay et al. 2006). A diet rich in natural antioxidants is best recommended, with ample amounts of a variety of fruits and vegetables.

6.14. Ultra-endurance events and altitude training

Ultra-endurance events are an area of endurance exercise and sport which warrants special consideration for dietary antioxidant supplementation. These events attract significant numbers of competitors from both non-elite amateurs and professional endurance athletes. The most well-known of these extreme events is the ironman triathlon with a 4-km swim, 180-km bike, and a complete 42-km marathon (Knez et al., 2007; Turner et al. 2011). Research investigating the effect of full and half-ironman triathlons on oxidative stress markers found that at rest, the ultra-endurance athletes had lower levels compared with relatively inactive controls (Knez et al. 2007), but post-competition elevations showed a significant inflammatory response. These athletes had relatively higher levels of erythrocyte antioxidant enzymes at rest but decreased in post-race enzymes that suggest a lack of antioxidant defense mechanisms. Oxidative stress levels may remain elevated following a sustained physical activity for many days. In an Ironman triathlon race, Neubauer et al. (2008) observed improvements in a variety of oxidative stress markers; after the event, these markers had taken five days to return to baseline (Neubauer et al. 2008).

The athletes taking antioxidant supplements may have higher levels of oxidative stress than age-matched, relatively inactive control subjects after half or full iron man triathlon competitions (Knez et al. 2007). Similarly, vitamin E (α-tocopherol) supplementation, two months before an ironman case, caused higher elevations of oxidative stress in post-race markers than placebo (Nieman et al. 2004). Another research investigating the impact of ultra-marathon swimming on oxidative stress (Kabasakalis et al. 2011) found no significant difference between pre-and post-race markers of oxidative stress, possibly due to the low-intensity nature of this activity compared to that studied in other sports which are at a higher average percentage of peak VO2. Another study investigating oxidative stress factors in response to swimmers ' training activities found that pre-and post-training flavonoid-based juice supplements did not reduce oxidative stress after exercise despite higher rates of oxidative stress compared with inactive controls (Knab et al. 2013).

The impact of altitude training requires special attention since altitude exposure can increase the production of oxidative stress irrespective of the duration or amount of exercise (Bakonyi and Radak 2004; Pialoux et al. 2009a, b). Therefore, it seems possible that during this period of heightened oxidative stress, increasing the supply of antioxidants would improve health, and possibly exercise. Studies were conducted using the altitude exposure method called' sleep high, exercise low.' Endurance training with intermittent resting hypoxia resulted in lower rates of antioxidant plasma resting without hypoxic exposure, with little change in the control group (Pialoux et al. 2009b). The restorative hypoxia community also reported a greater rise in post-training oxidative stress markers. Training with the added hypoxia tends to cause an increase in the production of free radicals, which depletes the body's antioxidant ability. The increased intake of antioxidants should help maintain antioxidant levels during this period. The loss in the hypoxia population did not return to baseline levels after two weeks of recovery (Pialoux et al. 2009a), indicating a more sustained impact on antioxidant concentrations. Other studies reported only a small difference in markers of oxidative stress in the supplemented population after two weeks of moderate-intensity exercise at high altitude (Subudhi et al. 2004). Amid prolonged submaximal cycling (55 percent VO2 max), the concentration of oxidative stress factors did not improve in this study. The increased oxidative stress caused by altitude exposure can play a significant role in adaptation, and dampening this effect with antioxidant supplementation can potentially impede adaptation.

Antioxidants can reduce the possible oxidative stress produced by high volume and intensity of endurance training. However, it is not absolutely clear whether increased oxidative stress triggered by training is, in fact, detrimental to the athlete. Further research is warranted by the degree to

238

which an increase in free radical production during high training loads influences the signaling required for adaptations to training. When solving these issues, athletes should seek advice from their health care practitioner(s) on antioxidant supplements that should assess individual requirements in terms of underlying health, nutritional diets, and training loads.

There's some evidence that increased dietary antioxidants change the course of the disease in diseases with an inflammatory etiology. Diets that increase fruit and/or vegetable intake (and therefore high in dietary antioxidants) are likely to have a number of unknown beneficial biological activities that are not measurable or observable. Further research is needed to decide whether nutritional approaches that help the disability groups in the general community, such as those with asthma, are transferred directly to hard-working but otherwise healthy endurance sportsmen.

Mixed antioxidant-rich diets can be safer than antioxidant supplementation and may offer greater benefits. Higher antioxidant intakes may help maintain a normal antioxidant / antioxidant balance. Supplementation with antioxidants can benefit endurance athletes undertaking extremely high levels of training, either living and/or exercising at moderate to high altitudes or participating in ultra-endurance competitions.

6.15. Athlete's guide to fighting inflammation

Exercising intensively triggers the release of substances known as free radicals. Free radicals can cause damage to the cells, loss of muscle function, and cause an inflammatory response. Eating antioxidant-rich foods and omega-3s helps protect the cell membranes from damage caused by these free radicals. Both nutrients contribute to the development and healing of damaged tissue and can help improve short- and long-term recovery from intense exercise.

6.16. Foods that fight inflammation

Vegetables-Rich in vitamins & antioxidants such as vitamins A, C, flavonoids, and carotenoids, vegetables are no brainer to help fight inflammation. Many of the richest sources include bell peppers, tomatoes, green leafy vegetables such as, but are not limited to, kale, spinach, and collard greens, beets, mushrooms (also high in vitamin D), broccoli, and sweet potatoes.

Berries–Research has shown that, before and after intense exercise, athletes who eat berries experience decreased inflammation and oxidant stress. The berries contain many antioxidants, including anthocyanins, vitamin C, and resveratrol. Add a variety to your diet, including blueberries, strawberries, goji berries, raspberries, and blackberries.5 Egg yolks–yolks are rich in vitamins including vitamins A, C, lutein, and zeaxanthin. While egg white omelets are often mistaken for being a "healthier" option, actually, the yolks you want are the ones. On all of those foods, you miss eating only the whites.

Whole grains–Because of their high fiber content, whole grains such as quinoa, brown rice, and oats can help protect against inflammation. Spices-Some spices, such as ginger or turmeric, contain anti-inflammatory compounds. Apply certain herbs to your dishes along with garlic or add a pinch to your smoothies.

Seeds-Seeds like flax and chia are high in fiber and omega-3 fatty acids. Baseball players-keep eating those sunflower seeds in the dugout! They're high in vitamin E and essential fatty acids.

Nuts–Rich in good antioxidants like vitamin E and anti-inflammatory fatty acids like omega-3, nuts should be a staple in your response to inflammation. Find a variety that includes almonds, walnuts, cashews, and pistachios.

Fatty fish–Fatty fish such as salmon, mackerel, herring, sardines, and albacore tuna are all high in omega-3 fatty acids. Although I always recommend food always but if you don't eat enough of these omega-3 rich foods in your diet, then you need to take an additional supplement, make sure you use a safe and approved drug. Search for the "NSF Certified for Sport" tag and ask a dietitian before beginning any new supplement.

The Tart Cherry Juice-Cherries are extremely rich in antioxidants. This concentrated cherry juice has been shown to reduce inflammation.

Citrus fruits–Citrus fruits are rich in protein, flavonoids, and vitamin C and can help combat inflammation and strengthen the immune system. Apply more citrus fruits like bananas, lemons, limes, and grapefruits to your diet.

Avocados–These "fruits" have anti-inflammatory effects, high in monounsaturated fats, vitamin E & C, and fiber. They are an excellent replacement for highly saturated fat spreads, such as mayonnaise or butter, on bread and sandwiches.

6.17. Foods to avoid

Refined starches such as pasta, white bread, and rice rapidly break down into sugar during the digestive process, which in turn may lead to inflammation, especially in high quantities. Inflammation can also lead to excessive amounts of added sugar such as glucose, fructose, molasses, a concentrate of fruit juice, high syrup of fructose corn, and syrup, to name a few. Consider raising the amount of fried, canned food that you consume, including cakes, crackers, cookies, and cereals. If sugar and flour are the first two ingredients, then pass it on and look for a better alternative.

In addition, **high intakes of trans and saturated fats may cause inflammation.** Monitor the intake of red meat and processed meat since they occur to be higher in saturated fat. Hydrogenated and "Partially Hydrogenated" (Trans Fat) are the most common in fried foods, snack foods, and sweets such as pastries, cookies, candies, and crackers. Read the ingredients, Mark. If the ingredient "partially hydrogenated" is listed, skip it.

Alcohol in moderation, mainly red wine due to its antioxidant content, can indeed be a good thing. But, going well beyond this "moderation" stage (i.e., no more than one women's drink, two men's drinks) could actually do more harm than good to your body.

6.18. Meal planning tips

Incorporating the foodstuffs described above can help to combat inflammation. Here are a few simple ideas/recipes which will help you put it into a meal plan.

Breakfast- Make a 2-egg omelet with peppers, onions, spinach, and mushrooms, or put it all together at the Casserole Market Breakfast from this farmer. Have a large bowl of fried berries. For athletes requiring additional calories, provide a side of oats with walnuts on top.

Lunch & Dinners- Take advantage of a grilled or broiled fish filet like salmon, lean protein like a chicken breast, or plant-based protein like quinoa bed lentils or brown rice. Finish with a heaping cup of green vegetables like broccoli or kale, season the platter with garlic, ginger or turmeric. To add some extra calories and healthy fats, chop up half an avocado and sprinkle the sesame or pumpkin seeds on top. Then render this Burrito Bowl with a Recipe.

Snacks- Enjoy fresh fruits and veggies like bananas, onions, carrots, or cucumbers eaten with a blended nut. Then dip apple slices into peanut butter than almond butter. Have a slice of whole-grain bread spread on top with almond butter, berries and flax seeds or mix in a smoothie with a variety of fruits and vegetables. Enjoy a glass of cherry juice, or make it into a smoothie-like your milk.

6.19. Reducing inflammation and Promoting recovery in athletes

Do you know inflammation is a normal part of the workout? Inflammation naturally occurs after a hard workout to help athletes heal muscles, and athletes can improve and adapt to more challenging workouts as the training continues.

Sleep well! Nonetheless, too much inflammation can become a problem that results from too many hard workouts with insufficient attention to recovery nutrition, adequate sleep, and unhealthy diets, and can have a negative impact on sports performance and impair immunity, which can lead to days off from practice or competition. Many athletes can turn to non-steroidal anti-inflammatory drugs (NSAIDs), such as ibuprofen, to decrease inflammation and reduce pain, but these drugs have been linked with stomach damage, and may potentially impede training adaptations that help athletes recover fast.

Soreness is part of daily training, but rather than popping up NSAIDs, with the following healthy diet and rest strategies put more focus on recovery and inflammation-fighting: make sleep a priority! The muscles rest and regenerate during sleep, and poor sleep can increase inflammation in the body. Increasing sleep and/or napping to a minimum of 8 hours can improve performance, mood, decrease tiredness, and improve reaction times and concentration.

Remove refined carbohydrates such as white rice and white bread, soda, French fries, and other processed foods such as crispy fried chicken, chips,pizza, and frozen fruit cakes, which may cause inflammation.

Add extra products to your plate by eating more antioxidant-containing fruits and vegetables, and phytochemicals that combat inflammation. Include anti-inflammatory foods in your daily diet, especially during periods of heavy training, such as tart cherry juice, turmeric, and fish oil.

Boost your consumption of healthy fats by snacking on walnuts, almonds, peanuts, flax seeds, using olive oil as a dressing on salads, and eating fatty fish like salmon and tuna for your protein for few meals a week to reduce inflammation.

Reducing or avoiding alcohol— over-consumption of alcohol can cause inflammation and disrupt sleep, which can be detrimental to long-term health together.

Eat enough calories to compensate for your physical activity and ensure the right amount of carbohydrates, protein, and healthy fats (macronutrients) is ingested. Not eating enough calories will increase the stress hormones, leaving athletes unable to fight off inflammation and heal properly after a hard workout.

Taking the holidays off! Rest days following intense workouts are an integral part of a training routine that helps athletes recover and make the next practice or match even better. Athletes who are running down, like they can't recover from their last practice/competition or see improvements in their performance, should speak to their coach about their training and take a look at their choice of diet and lifestyle to see where they can improve.

A sports dietitian will work with your workout schedule and current diet to help you achieve your goals for success this season by developing a nutrition plan that will help you perform better and get stronger through this season.

Chapter 7: Dietary Factors that have an impact on Inflammation Related to obesity

Diet is a key factor in controlling immune responses. There is considerable evidence that malnutrition is contributing to immune suppression because of a vulnerability to infection. On the other hand, over-nutrition leads to immune-activities, due to a susceptibility to an inflammatory disorder. Hence an optimal diet is needed for a healthy immune balance.

7.1. Carbohydrate

Carbohydrates are a significant source of dietary energy and can be measured using the GI and GL values. GI is a food classification based on their postprandial reaction to blood glucose, and a carbohydrate quality calculation. GL is a metric measuring both the amount and strength of the dietary carbohydrates. Large cross-sectional studies have demonstrated an association of GI / GL and inflammatory cytokines in the diet. In the Women's Health Research (n=13.187, > 45 years of age), the large quintiles of dietary GL and GI were significantly related to high blood levels of C-reactive protein (CRP). Similarly, in Dutch research (n=974, 42-87 years old), the highest quintile of dietary GI and GL was positively correlated with blood levels of CRP (p<0.05). In addition, the Nurse Health Survey (n=902, aged 30-55) and the follow-up survey of health professionals (n=532, aged 40-75)[39] found that a high GI or GL diet was significantly associated with low plasma adiponectin levels (p<0.05). The high levels of CRP and low levels of adiponectin in the blood are characterized as a low-grade inflammatory disorder associated with obesity. Ironically, inflammatory cytokine (CRP, TNF-α, and IL-6) randomized clinical trials did not exhibit a relationship between a high GI or GL diet. Nevertheless, 30 percent of the energy restriction in the high GL showed a decrease in serum CRP concentration in healthy overweight adults (n=34, 24-42 years old). Several detailed observational research found a positive correlation between a high GI/GL diet and inflammatory markers; however, the intervention studies could not convincingly support this association.

7.2. Dietary Fat

A high-fat diet induces excessive body fat accumulation, which affects the immune system. A variety of different fatty acids, including polyunsaturated (PUFA), saturated, and trans-fatty acids, have been examined for their effects on inflammatory conditions. Joffe et al. recently reviewed the effects of dietary fatty acids on gene expression and on the development of TNFα andIL-6.

PUFA omega-6 (n-6) PUFA and omega-3 (n-3) PUFA families are precursors of eicosanoids which play an important role in the immune response. Cross-sectional studies have identified the n-3 PUFA (eicosatetraenoic acid[EPA] and docosahexaenoic acid[DHA]) anti-inflammatory activity. The Nurses' Health Study I (n=727, aged 43-69) and the Attica Survey (n=3,042, aged 18-89) found that the consumption of n-3 fatty acids or fish is inverted to inflammatory biomarkers (CRP, IL-6, and TNF-α) (p<0.05). Interventional research (n=30, mean age 60 years) also reported that supplementation of fish oil (14 g / d of fish oil for five weeks) in healthy postmenopausal women decreased blood CRP andIL-6 levels.

Trans and saturated FA Observational and interventional research indicate a clear correlation between trans-or saturated FA and immune response. According to the Nurses ' Health Research I Cohort (n=730, 43-69 years of age), the highest quintile of trans-FAs intake was associated with high levels of CRP andIL-6 compared with the lowest quintile. In a randomized crossover trial (n=50), replacing trans-FAs (8%) with a high-fat diet (39% of fat) essentially increased blood levels of CRP and IL-6 (p<0.05). Likewise, replacing trans-FAs (< 7%) with a standard diet (30% of fat) increased the levels of IL-6 (as well as the levels of TNF-α but not CRP) in subjects with mild hypercholesterolemia.

7.3. Vegetable, fruits, and other nutrients

Numerous cross-sectional studies and some observational studies have documented an inverse correlation between high rates of vegetable and fruit consumption, either in combination or alone, and CRP. The Boston Puerto Rican Health research (n=1,159, 45-75 years of age) also found that variable fruit intake associated inversely with blood CRP levels. In addition, Salas-Salvadó et al. (n=772, 55-80 years of age) and Freese et al.

(n=77, 19-52 years of age) didn't show any link with inflammatory markers (adiponectin, CRP, IL-6, intercellular adhesion molecule-1[ICAM-1], vascular cell adherence molecule-1[VCAM-1]) between a vegetable and fruit-rich diet. Morand et al. (n=24, mean age 56) found that a single fruit supplement (500 mL of orange juice/d over four weeks) did not affect the levels of CRP, IL-6, ICAM-1, and VCAM-1.

Other Nutrients: Several vitamins and minerals have been shown to have beneficial effects on oxidative stress and immune responses. The association of vitamins and minerals with inflammatory marker levels (CRP, TNF-α, and IL-6) has been consistently demonstrated by cross-sectional and interventional research.

Vitamin A: Overweight or obese participants frequently reported lower plasma carotenoids due to the high proportion of carotenoids found as lipid-soluble compounds in adipose tissue. The Women's Health Study (n=2,895, aged around 45 years) reported higher plasma α-and β-carotene concentrations associated with low plasma CRP rates.

Vitamin C, in general, has beneficial effects on immunity. Aasheim et al. demonstrated that low plasma vitamin C levels were substantially associated with elevated levels of CRP in subjects with severe obesity (62 men and 106 women aged 19-59). Block et al. (n=216) supplemented vitamin C (515 mg / d over eight weeks) in stable smokers. They observed that supplementation with vitamin C significantly reduced levels of blood CRP (24 percent, $p<0.05$). In comparison, Fumeron et al.[58]

251

(n=42, aged 18-80) confirmed that vitamin C supplementation (750 mg / d for eight weeks) did not change blood levels of CRP.

Magnesium (Mg): Mg intake was inverted to dose-dependent levels of CRP, IL-6, and TNF-α-R2 in the Women's Health Study (n=3,713, 50-79 years of age), following adjustment for multiple variables, including dietary fiber, fat, meat, and vegetables. Guerrero-Romero and Rodríguez-Morán showed that low serum Mg levels were independently linked to elevated CRP concentration in non-diabetic, non-hypertensive obese subjects (n=371).

Flavonoids: A subclass of polyphenolic biological compounds, flavonoids are present in plant-derived vegetables, nuts, spices, chocolate, tea, and red wine. Several intervention studies have demonstrated strong antioxidant properties of flavonoids; however, their inflammatory and immune-regulatory effects are less clear. The Nurses ' Health Study (n=2,115, 43-70 years of age) found that low levels of pro-inflammatory biomarkers(IL-18 andsVCAM-1) were correlated with a diet rich in flavonoids (flavones, flavanones, and full flavonoids). The U.S. recently The Department of Agriculture (USDA, 2006) (n=8,335, around 19 years old) confirmed that high dietary intake of flavonoids was inversely associated with plasma concentration of CRP ($p<0.05$). A randomized, parallel controlled study (n=120, 40-74 years of age) found that the supplementation of bilberry juice (300 mL / d for three weeks) decreased plasma levels of pro-inflammatory cytokines (TNF-α, IL-6, and-8, with no changes in CRP). Karlsen et al. recently reported that the use of bilberry juice (330 mL / d for four weeks) significantly reduced plasma levels of pro-inflammatory cytokines (TNF-α, IL-6, and IL-15) and CRP in CVD-risk subjects (n=62, 34-68 years of age). By contrast, a double-blind, placebo-controlled crossover study (n=14, 35-53 years old) found that marine buckthorn flavanol extract supplementation for four weeks did not reduce CRP levels ($p<0.05$).

7.4. Phytoestrogens, probiotics, and prebiotics

Phytoestrogens are plant origin compounds found in a wide variety of foods, beans, nuts, and grains. It's assumed that phytoestrogens have anti-inflammatory properties. A diet of naturally isoflavone-enriched pasta, aglycones (33 mg / d), decreased plasma CRP concentrations significantly in a randomized, controlled study. When the subjects were changed back to a traditional diet (n=62, mean age 58.2 years), plasma CRP levels returned to baseline. Meanwhile, in a study of healthy postmenopausal women, the supplementation of soy isoflavone (genistein at 54 or 40 mg / d) for six months did not affect rates of CRP (n=30, 50-60 years of age, and n=80, mean age 49.5 years). Similarly, in a study of obese postmenopausal women, soy isoflavone supplementation for six months had no impact on plasma CRP concentration (n=50, mean age 58). There are studies that the supplementation of phytoestrogen has beneficial effects on inflammatory markers, but the results are contradictory.

Probiotics are living micro-organisms that provide a health benefit to their host. Orally ingested probiotic bacteria can modulate the immune system; however, different probiotic strains may have different immune-modulatory effects. In a randomized, double-blind, placebo-controlled trial, in healthy subjects (n=30, 23-43 years of age), the combination of Lactobacillus gasseri and Lactobacillus coryniformis with Staphylococcus thermophilus had no effect on serum TNF-α or IL-12 concentrations. Comparisons with L were made by Kekkonen et al. Bifidobacterium ssp animalis. Rhamnosus lactis Bb12, and propionibacterium freudenreichii ssp. Shermanii JS during three weeks in healthy subjects (n=81, ages 23-58). There was no effect on serum levels of TNF-α, IL-6, IL-10or IFN-ÿ but a reduced level of CRP in the L. Group of rhamnosus supplementation. Although it has been shown that probiotics have beneficial effects on inflammatory markers, further studies are needed to arrive at the definitive results.

Prebiotics are non-digestible elements of food that provide a health benefit to the host associated with the regulation of microbiota in the gut. The IL-6 mRNA expression decreased by oligofructose, a common form of prebiotics, supplementation (8 g / d for three weeks) in the elderly (n=19, mean 85 years of age). By contrast, oligofructose supplementation (1.95-3.9 g / d for 12 weeks) had no effect on IL-6 or TNF-α plasma levels in poorly nourished elderly subjects (mean age 70 years). Although a convincing correlation between a prebiotic supplementation and inflammatory markers has been shown by a few observational studies, drawing this beneficial association is currently premature.

7.5. 1,200 Calorie Anti-inflammatory diet plan for weight loss

The anti-inflammatory diet is about consuming more of the foods that help to reduce inflammation in the body while reducing the foods that tend to increase inflammation, thereby helping to fight inflammatory conditions. The diet includes many colorful fruits and vegetables, high-fiber legumes and whole grains, healthy fats (such as those found in salmon, nuts and olive oil) and antioxidant-rich herbs, spices and tea, thus minimizing processed foods made with unhealthy trans fats, refined carbohydrates (such as white flour and added sugar), and too much sodium.

In this healthy 1200-calorie meal plan, they put together the principles of anti-inflammatory eating to offer a week of tasty, wholesome meals and snacks, plus meal-prep tips to set you up for a good week ahead to achieve weight loss.

As inflammation can be caused by many other factors in addition to food, such as low rates of exercise, stress, and lack of sleep, it can also help prevent inflammation by incorporating healthy lifestyle habits into your daily routine. Combine this balanced meal plan with daily physical exercise (aimed at moderate intensity for 2 1/2 hours a week), stress-relieving exercises (such as yoga, meditation or something that works best for you), and a good night's sleep every night (at least 7 hours a night), to

255

get the most anti-inflammatory benefits. Whether you're working actively to minimize inflammation or just searching for a balanced diet plan, this 7-day anti-inflammatory meal plan will help.

Meal prep for a week

At the beginning of the week, a little meal prep will set you up for healthy-eating success.

Prepare the Vegan Superfood Buddha Bowls for Days 2, 3, 4, and 5 to have lunch. Refrigerate the bowls and separate dressing for up to 4 days. Avoid until you are ready to eat, adding avocado to avoid browning.

Make the Tahini Dip with Turmeric-Ginger to have snacks throughout the week.

Day 1:

Foods that contain high omega-3 fatty acids, such as salmon, sardines, and albacore tuna, have been shown to reduce levels of inflammation. Try to include at least two portions of 3-ounce fish rich in omega-3 fatty acids each week.

Breakfast (287 calories): 1 serving overnight Blueberry-Banana Oats, 1 cup of green tea

Lunch (325 calories): 1 serving Green Salad with Edamame & Beets

Snack (117 calories): 2 Tbsp. Turmeric ginger tahini dip. 1 carrot. Cut that into sticks

Dinner (442 calories): 1 serving Walnut-Rosemary Crusted Salmon, 1 serving Roasted Squash & Apples with Dried Cherries

Daily Totals: 1,202 calories, 57 g of protein, 131 g of carbohydrate, 30 g of fiber, 54 g of fat, 1,520 mg of sodium.

Day 2:

Anti-inflammatory bonus: An antioxidant, vitamin C has anti-inflammatory properties because it helps to decrease dangerous free radical cells that can cause inflammation. Studies prove that people with diets high in vitamin C have lower levels of the C-reactive protein inflammatory marker as well as a lower risk of inflammatory diseases, such as gout and heart disease. Today's Raspberry-Kefir Power Smoothie provides 45 percent of Vitamin C's recommended daily value!

Breakfast (249 calories): 1 portion Raspberry-Kefir Power Smoothie A.M.

Snack (28 calories): 1/3 cup of blueberries

Lunch (381 calories): 1 serving Vegan Superfood Buddha Bowl P.M.

Snack (9 calories): 1/2 cup of sliced cucumber flavored with a pinch of salt and pepper each.

Dinner (393 calories): 1 serving Indian-Spiced Cauliflower & Chickpea Salad, 5 ounces of water (drained) Bottom tuna salad.

Evening snack (156 calories): 1 ounce of dark chocolate

Daily total: 1,215 calories, 70 g of protein, 143 g of carbohydrate, 35 g of fiber, 47 g of fat, 1.054 mg of sodium

Day 3:

Anti-inflammatory bonus: Anthocyanins are strong antioxidant compounds found in dark blue fruits and vegetables, red and purple, as well as red wine. Research suggests that anthocyanins parts a role in decreasing signs of inflammation, which can reduce cancer risk and heart disease. Keep frozen berries on hand to give your morning smoothies or oatmeal an anti-inflammatory boost, so you can get the benefits even when they're not in season!

Breakfast (263 calories): 1 cup of low-fat plain Greek yogurt 1 1/2 (Blueberries 1/4 cup sliced walnuts 1 cup green tea Top walnuts and blueberries yogurt.

Snack (42 calories): 2/3 cup raspberries

 Lunch (381 calories): 1 portion Vegan Superfood Buddha Bowl P.M.

Snack (117 calories): 2 Tbsp Turmeric ginger tahini.

Dinner (409 calories): 1 portion Superfood Chopped Salad with Salmon & Creamy Garlic Dressing

Daily Totals: 1,212 calories 77 g of protein, 97 g of carbohydrate, 28 g of fiber, 63 g of fat, 813 mg of sodium.

Day 4:

Anti-inflammatory bonus: moderate intake of dark chocolate and cacao will reduce inflammatory markers and improve heart health. Cocoa is rich in flavanol quercetin, a potent antioxidant that protects our cells, and a major component of the anti-inflammatory diet is dark chocolate. Incorporate the darkest chocolate one 1-ounce square a day that you will find to maximize benefits.

Breakfast (222 calories): 1 portion Cocoa-Chia Pudding with Raspberries

A.M. Snack (109 calories): Half cup low-fat Greek yogurt with 1/4 cup of blueberries

Lunch (381 calories): 1 portion Vegan Superfood Buddha Bowl

P.M. Snack (9 calories): 1/2 cup sliced cucumber Pinch of salt Pinch of pepper Dinner (472 calories) 1 serving Stuffed Sweet Potato with Hummus Dressing

Daily Total: 1,191 calories, 56 g protein, 168 g carbohydrate, 49 g fiber, 39 g fat, 1,100 mg sodium

Day 5:

Anti-inflammatory bonus: Probiotics such as those present in kimchi, yogurt, kefir, and kombucha help support healthy intestines. Research shows a healthy gut is enhancing our immune systems, helping to maintain a healthy weight, and reducing inflammation. Always make sure to include prebiotics, which are indigestible plant fibers found in foods such as garlic, onions, and whole grains, which help to provide fuel for good bacteria to improve our gut health.

Breakfast (249 calories): Raspberry-Kefir Power Smoothie

A.M. Snack (2 calories): 1 cup of green tea

Lunch (381 calories): 1 Vegan Superfood Buddha Bowl

P.M. Snack (58 calories): 1 tablespoon Turmeric-Ginger Tahini Dip with 3/4 cup sliced cucumber

Dinner (414 calories): 1 portion Korean Steak, Kimchi & Cauliflower Rice Bowl Evening

Snack (120 calories): 5 ounces of red wine

Daily Totals: 1,224 calories, 57 g of protein, 112 g of carbohydrates, 28 g of sugar, 53 g of fat, 1,067 mg of sodium.

Day 6:

Anti-inflammatory bonus: Any form of arthritis, an inflammatory joint condition, which is often treated with a mixture of an anti-inflammatory diet and prescription medication, affects more than 20 percent of U.S. adults. The best anti-inflammatory diet for arthritis involves a lot of magnesium studies, which indicates that it reduces inflammation and helps to maintain joint cartilage. Many Americans don't get enough magnesium, so make sure to include plenty of nuts, legumes, whole grains, and seeds to ensure adequate intake.

Breakfast (249 calories): 1 serving Raspberry-Kefir Power Smoothie

A.M. Snack (157 calories): 12 walnut halves

Lunch (325 calories): 1 serving Green Salad with Edamame & Beets

P.M. Snack (78 calories): 1/2 ounce of dark chocolate

Dinner (401 calories): 1 serving Hummus-Crusted Chicken 1 serving Blistered Broccoli with Garlic and Chiles Meal-Prep Tip: Cook and save the extra chicken for lunch. You will require two cups of cooked chicken, chopped.

Daily Total: 1,209 calories, 73 g of protein, 94 g of carbohydrate, 28 g of fruit, 63 g of fat, 1,245 mg of sodium.

Day 7:

Anti-inflammatory bonus: A diet rich in fiber would have a lower glycemic index, a measure of how our blood sugars are affected by food.

260

Fiber is slowly digested, which keeps us full and enhances the regulation of blood sugar. Additional bonus-eating food is lower on the glycemic index that helps lower levels of C-reactive protein, which is a marker for inflammation. A balanced anti-inflammatory diet provides a total of 28 grams of fiber every day.

Breakfast (292 calories): 1 serving Cocoa-Chia Pudding with Raspberries 1 Turmeric Latte

A.M. Snack (42 calories): 1/2 cup of blueberries

Lunch (350 calories): 1 serving Avocado Egg Salad Sandwiches

P.M. Snack (116 calories): 15 unsalted almonds

Dinner (448 calories): 1 serving single-pot Garlicky Shrimp & Spinach 1 cup of cooked quinoa

Daily Totals: 1,209 calories, 62 g of protein, 128 g of carbohydrate, 32 g of fiber, 55 g fat, 1,362 mg sodium.

Chapter 8: The Anti-Inflammatory Lifestyle

Inflammation is one of the natural ways the body defends itself. This involves multiple chemical reactions that help fight off infections, increase blood flow to places where healing is needed, and create pain as a sign that something is wrong with the body. Unfortunately, as any process in the body, one can possess too much of a good thing.

Inflammation is sometimes equivalent to an acid. There is no doubt that fire keeps us dry, protected, and covered in limited quantities, but it can be dangerous when there is too much fire, or when fire gets out of control. But that doesn't have to be high for damage to cause a fire. It is now evident that low-grade chronic or recurrent inflammation, which is below the level of pain, can contribute to many chronic problems of health and can become a disease itself. This low-grade inflammation can prevent proper tissue healing and can also start killing healthy cells in the lungs, muscles, joints, and other parts of the body.

Too much inflammation is associated with a range of medical conditions. Some of these include:

• Alzheimer's disease

• Asthma

• Obesity

• Chronic obstructive lung disease (emphysema and bronchitis)

• Chronic pain

- Type 2 diabetes

- Heart disease

- Inflammatory intestinal disease (Crohn's disease or ulcerative colitis)

- Stroke

- Body-attacked disorders such as rheumatoid arthritis, lupus, or scleroderma.

The most famous test is to check your blood for the amount of C-reactive protein (hsCRP).

How to prevent or reduce excessive inflammation: In order to reduce inflammation, people often take medicines. Drugs such as ibuprofen and aspirin can change the body's chemical reactions but are not without side effects. Research has shown that lifestyle choices can also minimize inflammation; our choices can affect the degree to which we have inflammation within our bodies. Adapting to a healthy diet as well as other healthy lifestyle habits can have a dramatic effect on inflammatory levels.

8.1. What is an Anti-inflammatory lifestyle?

The anti-inflammatory lifestyle includes the following features:

- Consuming anti-inflammatory food

- No smoking

- Reducing alcohol intake

- Adequate exercise

- Getting enough sound sleep

- Stress management

- Weight management

8.2. Eating to reduce inflammation

Everything we eat can affect inflammation, and certain foods are more likely to reduce the effects of pain and other illnesses. Approximate 60 percent of chronic diseases could be avoided by a healthy diet, including many of the health problems listed above.

2 Consuming the right foods can not only mitigate the onset of inflammation in the first place but can also help to reduce and resolve chronic inflammations.

Anti-inflammatory way of eating: Reducing inflammation is not one-size-fits-all. A number of people would do it differently. The traditional Mediterranean diet, influenced by some Mediterranean basin nations, is one of the most researched examples of an anti-inflammatory way of eating.

Those who regularly follow a Mediterranean-like diet have significantly lower inflammatory levels compared to other less balanced approaches to food.

The Mediterranean diet protects against many chronic conditions, including cardiovascular disease, type 2 diabetes mellitus, Alzheimer's and Parkinson's disease, and some cancers.

The Mediterranean diet is just 1 example of a traditional diet and seems to be the best-researched traditional diet in the world. Most traditional diets are healthier than current popular diets, as they concentrate on eating organic, unprocessed foods, shared with family and friends. The specificities of the Mediterranean Diet that vary from study to study, but these are often common elements.

Usually (though not exclusively), the **Mediterranean diet** is a plant-based diet, rich in fresh fruits and vegetables, whole grain cereals, and legumes. It advocates nuts, seeds, and olive oil as fat sources and needs moderate intakes of fish and shellfish, eggs, white meat, and fermented dairy products (cheese and yogurt), and relatively small amounts of sweets and red and processed meats. It is possible that the diet as a whole, rather than individual contents, leads to good results. The various components work together to reduce the inflammation and bring about beneficial effects in the body.

Several primary aspects of the Mediterranean diet include:
- Relatively high fat intake (30-50 percent of total daily calories) o Usually from monounsaturated fatty acids (mainly olive oil) o Saturated fats make up less than 8 percent of calories.
- Heavy fruit and vegetable intake
- Low fiber consumption (32 g / day)
- High in easily digested carbohydrates (i.e., low glycemic load). For more details, please see Managing Better Health Dietary Carbohydrates. The Mediterranean diet is just 1 example of a typical diet pattern. In general, traditional diet patterns are safe, anti-inflammatory patterns because they do not contain processed foods.

8.3. Consuming more anti-inflammatory food

Eat a vibrant, well-balanced diet with lots of vegetables and fruit: Diets high in fruits and vegetables that provide essential antioxidants and phytochemicals with good anti-inflammatory nutrients; some beneficial plant substances, called phytochemicals, include brightly colored fruits and vegetables, usually green, orange, black, red, and purple. Most of these compounds have antioxidant properties that can assist in minimizing inflammation. Studies show a diet high in fruits and vegetables is beneficial. Fruit and vegetables: The more you cook, the better you eat. A good target of a variety of vegetables and fruits, including dark green, brown, yellow, red, and legumes (beans and peas), is at least 4 1/2 cup-equivalents per day. Of sweet, "soft" vegetables like lettuce, and raw spinach, one cup counts as 1/2 cup-equivalent. One-half cup counts as an average of 1/2 cups for denser vegetables such as peas, green beans, or chopped sweet peppers. Insist on fruit over vegetables. Purple and red berries are particularly full of anti-inflammatory compounds, as are cruciferous vegetables such as broccoli, kale, cabbage, and cauliflower.

Increase the quantity of Omega-3 Fatty Acids: Foods containing long-chain omega-3 fatty acids such as cold-water fish (salmon, sardines, and tuna) are particularly suitable for decreasing inflammation. Typically found in plants, omega-3 fatty acids abundant in fatty fish, eicosapentaenoic acid (EPA) and docosahexaenoic acid (DHA) are more potent anti-inflammatory agents than alpha-linolenic acid (ALA) (2-3 servings of fatty fish such as salmon, mackerel, herring, lake trout, sardines and albacore tuna per week). ALA converts to EPA and then to

DHA, but less than 1 percent of the initial ALA is transformed into the physiologically active EPA and DHA.

For this reason, the ALA-rich flax oil is not as good as EPA and DHA for inflammation. Fish oil contains EPA and DHA (about 18% and 12% respectively) and is a good source of these essential fatty acids. Plant sources of omega-3s usually contain ALA, but now there are vegan supplements derived from algae that contain both EPA and DHA.

Consider adding fresh fish oil to your diet. 1 gm of fish oil contains approximately 0.5-1 gm of total omega-3, so aim 3-4 gm of fish oil per day or 5-4 gm for inflammatory treatments.

Improve intake of olive oil: extra virgin olive oil is an excellent choice when cooking, as it has been shown to be lower in blood pressure, LDL cholesterol, and inflammatory markers.

Pay attention to the oils in popular salad dressings and opt for olive oil where possible. Olive oil contains mainly monounsaturated fatty acids (not omega-3 or -6s) and comes in several grades; "pure' is the most processed,' virgin' has modest processing, and extra virgin olive oil (EVOO) is minimally processed and valued for its presence of many potent beneficial phytochemicals.

Cook well with "Fresh" and "Virgin." It is best not to cook with EVOO as heating it to a moderate temperature will reduce the phytochemical content by around 15 percent-25 percent, but the benefits of monounsaturated fatty acids remain. EVOO may be added after cooking or used for making salad dressings. Canola oil is a better option as a mainly monounsaturated oil, but it does not contain many of the beneficial olive oil phytochemicals, and less research is done to support its anti-inflammatory effects. Certain oils that are relatively high in monounsaturated fatty acids include almond, rice bran, and sesame oils, but they also contain moderate amounts of omega-6s.

Coconut oil: There is growing interest in cooking with coconut oil. Coconut oil is "heart-healthy" or not is currently under discussion. Coconut oil tends to increase more HDL-cholesterol (the "healthy" cholesterol) than LDL-cholesterol (the "poor" cholesterol), thereby leading to a more favorable cholesterol profile compared with butter. Therefore, in the case of traditional diets where coconut oil is consumed daily, this does not appear to cause damage.

This means which it is important to understand the rest of the diet, not just the oil itself. It is suggested that coconut oil, in the context of an unhealthy Western diet, can increase cardiovascular risk. In terms of inflammation, preliminary animal research suggests that extra virgin coconut oil may have anti-inflammatory properties, but there is still a lack of human research.

Using Tea and Other Spices: Spices such as ginger and turmeric contain other important anti-inflammatory compounds to improve those in your diet by drinking teas (green is a strong anti-inflammatory tea) and use those spices in your cooking.

8.4. Avoid inflammatory foods

Avoid trans-fatty acids: Trans fatty acids stimulate inflammation. Items that may contain trans-fats, also referred to as "hydrogenated oils," include margarine, deep-fried foods, and processed foods designed for long shelf life, such as crackers and packaged foods.

Restricted Refined Seed Vegetable Oils: Restrict seed oils (soybeans, corn, sunflower, grapes, cotton seeds, and wheat germ oils) and processed foods high in omega-6 fatty acids, and select sources of monounsaturated fatty acids, such as canola and olive oils, while increasing the intake of omega-3-rich foods (such as fatty cold water); The seed oils given above are not necessarily harmful in limited amounts. It's just that they're a lot of in the western diet.

The history story on omega-6 fatty acids Omega-6 fatty acids is abundant in the traditional western diet. These are found in high concentration in the conventional seed oils mentioned above, and hence in many processed foods (crackers, chips, fast foods). What effect omega 6 fatty acids have on inflammation and on chronic health conditions remains unclear. Recent research has suggested that there is too much interaction between these dietary fatty acids and body proinflammatory pathways. Nonetheless, more recent research suggests that omega-6 fatty acids may not directly increase inflammation, and may actually act in an anti-inflammatory manner, depending on other factors.

What is evident, however, is that omega-3 fatty acids, like those from cold-water fish, have anti-inflammatory, and thus beneficial health effects.

What can you think about it?

The evidence suggests that human beings evolved between omega-6 and omega-3 on a diet with an essential fatty acid ratio of about 1:1. The current western diets are in the range of around 10-25:1.

Yet ancient humans ate a lot fewer omega-6 than conventional fatty acids in America. Since seed oils are so widely used in most processed foods, the best way to reduce your omega-6 intake is by reducing processed foods in your diet.

All fatty acids omega-3 and-6 are essential nutrients in your diet, so you need some omega-6s, but you should limit them. Hence, focus on increasing the dietary omega-3s and reducing the dietary omega-6s while maintaining all essential dietary fats.

Reduce Saturated Fat Consumption: Recent evidence continues to indicate that food with high dietary saturated fat consumption in the context of an unhealthy Western diet is associated with low but increased risk of cardiovascular disease and low but increased rates of inflammation, especially for overweight and obese people.

Nonetheless, when reducing saturated fat, the emphasis on poly-and monounsaturated fats and particularly omega-3 fatty acids, rather than carbohydrates, is crucial. In the context of the whole diet the intake of the aforementioned anti-inflammatory foods leads to a positive synergistic effect.

• Regular dairy consumption Full-fat and non-fermented dairy products may have a small effect on increased inflammation, but overall, dairy products do not appear to increase inflammation. Moreover, fermented dairy products such as yogurt and Kiefer have a neutral or even positive effect on cardiovascular risk and inflammation. Consumption of dairy products, especially yogurt in regular amounts, may be learned. To be sure to minimize sugar intake, choose basic, unsweetened varieties.

Regulate the intake of red meat: Those consuming the most overall red meat remain at the highest risk of diabetes, cardiovascular disease, and multiple cancers. Recent evidence, however, suggests that the main culprit may be the processed red meat, such as hot dogs, sausages, and lunch meats.

Red meat is one of the good sources of protein, iron, and other micronutrients, but it can be a good substitute for poultry, eggs, and dairy as well as vegetable proteins (legumes) and grains. Pick unprocessed grass-fed sources that may have more desirable fatty-acid profiles if you eat red meat, pick lean cuttings, and trim visible fat. The World Cancer Research Fund recommends 12 to 18 ounces of red meat per week (three 6 oz servings or six 3 oz servings), cooked weight; 3 oz is about the size of a card deck. Avoid processed foods like bacon, salami, hot dogs, and sausages.

Giving Charring up: Food Charring is related to inflammation.

Reduce Blood Sugar: The body easily breaks down foods high in refined carbohydrates such as white flour, rice, bread, and refined sugar into simple sugars that are rapidly absorbed and can cause large spikes in the hormone insulin that promote inflammation. Better to limit or avoid such foods.

Eat low-GL: eat low-GL foods and meal plans (see Managing Better Health Carbohydrates).

Those include complex carbohydrates (such as unprocessed whole grains, starchy vegetables, and fruits), foods high in protein, fat, and fiber that help balance blood sugar and reduce the inflammatory effects of insulin. As complex carbohydrates are consumed in conjunction with high-fiber foods and healthy oils, carbohydrate degradation is delayed, and the overall glycemic load is that.

Consume More Fiber: Diets high in fiber aim to reduce inflammation.

Fiber helps slow the absorption of carbohydrates, helps to control blood sugar levels, and also helps to keep you full longer. Mechanisms by which fiber minimizes inflammation are not fully understood, but fiber promotes fat recycling in the body, and also attracts "clean" bacteria in the intestines that have a positive effect on inflammatory pathways. Complete, fiber-rich foods often contain several essential phytochemicals with anti-inflammatory properties.

The fiber target is 30 grams a day, or more. Get used to reading packaged food nutrition labels to help you find more fiber options for the products. Nevertheless, fiber is better derived from whole foods. Total fiber intake can be difficult to keep track of, but if you eat a healthy diet pattern like the Mediterranean diet, you usually get plenty of fiber. See the tips below for some safe ways to increase your fiber intake.

Ensure adequate Magnesium: (Mg) intake deficiency is associated with increased inflammation. Due to poor nutrition, Mg is under-consumed in the US, and it is estimated that 60 percent of Americans do not get enough. Dark green vegetables are an affluent source of Mg as well as legumes, nuts, seeds, and whole grains. The recommended dietary allowance (RDA) for Mg for females and males over age is 320 and 420 mg / d, respectively. It does not appear that consumption beyond that point gives any further benefit. One cup of spinach or Swiss chard contains about 150 mg; 1/4 C of pumpkin seed contains 190 mg; 1 Cup of black beans, 3/4 C of quinoa, and 1/4 C of cashew or sunflower seed contains about 120 mg, respectively.

Be patient: It takes some time for the anti-inflammatory eating to work. Try them for at least six weeks or longer. Eventually, it must become a natural way of eating in order to keep you safe over the long term.

Fiber Tips Change your carbohydrate sources to full-food carbohydrate sources such as starchy vegetables, legumes, whole grains, and fruits, keeping your glycemic load small.

One-half cup starchy vegetables (beets, corn, green peas, parsnips, winter squash, sweet potatoes, and pumpkin) contain around 2-4 grams of fiber. One medium apple contains 4 to 5 grams of fiber, and about 3.5 grams of fiber originates from a medium orange. Carbohydrates shape around a quarter of your plate.

The legumes: Eating at least one serving (1/2 cup) of legumes (beans and peas) every day can go a long way for gaining your target of fiber. A 1/2 cup of cooked lentils, garbanzo or black beans contains 6 to 9 grams of fiber. All beans are a good source of obtaining fiber and create a variety in your diet, add it to soups, and use pureed beans as dips and spreads (think hummus!). Start slow to prevent excessive gas and to bloat; the body eventually adapts.

Use whole grains over refined grains. Entire grains are treated minimally so that the whole grain remains intact. Whole grains contain oats, brown rice, quinoa, millet, barley, buckwheat, bulgur wheat, amaranth. 1/2 cup includes 2-4 grams of fiber
• Include and eat vegetables in each meal. One study indicated that when people ate a salad before the main meal, they consumed 23% more vegetables than those eating salad at mealtime, increased their fiber intake and lowered their calorie intake.

8.5. Tips to an anti-inflammatory lifestyle

Being healthy exercise has been shown to reduce inflammation, and people who get regular physical activity have lower levels of inflammation. Guidelines for physical activity include:
A cumulative goal of 150 minutes (30 minutes 5 days a week) of moderate aerobic physical activity such as tennis or walking, or 75 minutes (1 hour and 15 minutes a week) of intense physical activity.

Muscle-reinforcing workouts (such as weight training or resistance bands) of medium to high intensity on two days or more a week.

Get Enough Quality Sleep: Sound Sleep is one of the most important things people need to keep their minds and their bodies healthy. The Centers for Disease Control suggests that approximately 35 percent of US adults do not get the optimum 7 hours of sleep a night. People who do not get enough sleep or who have frequent interruptions or poor quality sleep are more likely to have more inflammation and also health problems such as type 2 diabetes and weight gain.

Manage stress: Stress exists in many ways, such as physical (hazard threat), mental (job or financial stress), and emotional (social rejection, isolation, or relationship stress).

Stress is a part of life and may change during life. If stress is overwhelming or if there is moderate ongoing stress that is not relieved, the body could lose its ability to respond healthily, resulting in increased inflammation that could harm our health. It can build the ability to manage stress. All of the above techniques— eating a healthy diet, getting active, and getting enough sleep — improve the ability of the body to deal with life stresses. Certain approaches like mind-body strategies like mind-based stress reduction (MBSR), progressive muscle relaxation (PMR), biofeedback, breathing exercises, yoga, and tai-chi can be useful.

Weight management: Inflammatory equilibrium in the body is caused by several factors. Some evidence indicates maintaining a healthy weight may be important for inflammation management. People who are obese, or who have excess abdominal weight, have a higher risk of inflammation than others. In particular, those located in the abdominal area, fat cells (known as adipocytes), develop and secrete compounds that can lead to inflammation. Fortunately, even a small weight loss of 10% of body weight can help to reduce inflammation. Aim of a healthy diet like a Mediterranean diet or an anti-inflammatory diet.

Description: Each of those lifestyle factors can aid in reducing inflammation. Bite off a convenient bit, and change one at a time. This will help improve and retain the ability to make changes. Trying to find a balance in your life, handling stress in a healthy way, being part of a community, spending time outside, doing exercise, sleeping well, and, most importantly, spending time with people you love is just as vital as eating food. You must feed yourself as a whole–mind, body, heart, and spirit.

Note: The recommendations here are detailed suggestions for a dietary plan, which can help to reduce inflammation. Individuals may have particular sensitivities to the food, which may contribute to inflammation.

Chapter 9: The inflammatory diet to avoid in order to cure various inflammatory diseases

The elimination diet is the eating program that omits a food or group of foods that are believed to cause an adverse food reaction, often referred to as "food intolerance." By avoiding certain foods for a period of time, and then re-introducing them during a "challenge" period, you will identify the foods that cause symptoms or make them worse. We also think of food reactions as a sudden allergic reaction, like a person getting an anaphylactic reaction to eating peanuts and swelling their throats.

However, there are several other ways our bodies react to foods that might not be so immediate and may or may not be correlated with an immune response. Food intolerances can be induced by various natural compounds found in foods (natural sugars or proteins) or by common food additives (such as natural and artificial colors, preservatives, antioxidants, and taste enhancers) that can trigger reactions via different mechanisms in the organism. The precise mechanisms involved in the different food reactions are still being discussed, and many studies may be unsuccessful in identifying the suspected culprit(s). Clinical experience has shown that a diet on elimination is one of the best resources for identifying food culprits and is very healthy as long as a variety of foods are still eaten containing all the nutrients needed.

9.1. Symptoms

Symptoms of food intolerance can vary widely. These can involve the stomach and abdominal swelling, headaches, hives, itching, and even vague signs of being unwell, such as flu and pains, extreme tiredness, or concentration problems. It is also known that certain foods and food groups intensify symptoms in people with specific illnesses, such as autoimmune disorders, migraines, irritable bowel syndrome, gastroesophageal reflux (GERD), and others. Symptoms and severity are special to the person. They are affected by different compounds in the food, a person's level of sensitivity, and how much those foods are consumed. By consuming the same food on a regular basis or eating different foods together or regularly with the same ingredient, the body may reach a threshold or tipping point where symptoms begin to develop.

Natural Food Substances: Only "healthy" foods contain a number of different chemicals that occur naturally, and for some people can be a concern. Substances similar in various foods, such as salicylates, amines, and glutamate, may cause different people symptoms. Providing information about the different categories of natural substances that may cause symptoms is beyond the scope of this handout, but this can be addressed with a practitioner who is comfortable working with removal diets (not all practitioners are).

Human variability: Because people are genetically unique, and each of us has various eating patterns, increasing human needs to focus on diets for elimination. The most successful way of finding out which foods can contribute to the symptoms is to remove the most offensive food or many foods and substances all at once. A healthcare practitioner can recommend that a particular plan be followed based on symptoms, typical dietary choices, and food cravings.

9.2. The Elimination Diet Steps

The Elimination Diet has four key steps:

Step 1

Planning Consult with your health care provider to find out which foods may cause problems. You will be asked to keep a diet log for a week, list the foods you consume, and keep track of the symptoms you have for the entire day. See the final page of this handout for a Food Diary Poster, which you can use.

A few main questions to ask yourself are helpful:

• Which foods do I eat the most often?

• What foods do I want?

• Which foods do I eat to "feel better"?

• Which foods would I have trouble giving up?

Sometimes these seem to be the most important things to look for and not eat. Make a list of issues of potential foods.

Depending on how many suspicious food culprits are avoided, the extent of the elimination diet can differ. It is possible to follow three different "levels" of food exclusion based on potential food culprits and the probability of adhering to the diet. The three levels are listed below in the Eliminating Diet Strategies section on page 6. First of all, it is helpful to consider choosing the approach that is the least restrictive in order to optimize successful adherence to the restrictions. Nevertheless, more rigorous methods are more effective in identifying cases that involve multiple culprits against food.

Are You Ready?

It is important to consider before beginning a diet on elimination, whether it is a good time to undergo these potentially large changes in diet. Do you have any planned stressful events or lifetime journeys? Do you have the money, will, and ability to create new cooking lists and menus?

Are you supported by family and friends for eating at home, at college, at restaurants, and other events? It will be important to remove the foods on your list entirely for 2-4 weeks, so if you somehow accidentally eat one of the foods, you'll have to start again. If you succeed the first time, it's going to be faster and easier.

Step 2

Make a list of foods to avoid depending on your planning, and be sure to avoid potential "hidden products" (see table 3).

Begin the elimination diet, and maintain the elimination diet for two to four weeks without exception.

Do not eat as a whole or as ingredients the foods excluded from other foods. For instance, if you avoid all dairy products, you need to check the

281

whey, casein, and lactose labels to avoid them as well. The step requires much discipline. Food labels should be very cautious. Be particularly careful when eating out, as you have less control over what's going into your food. If you make some mistake and eat something on the list, then you should start over again.

Most people notice their symptoms may get worse in the first week, especially during the first few days, before they begin to get better. If your symptoms escalate or become serious over a day or two, contact your health care practitioner.

Step 3

If your signs have not improved in two weeks, live for up to 4 weeks. If your symptoms have not better by the end of 4 weeks, leave the diet and start retrying this process with another combination of foods.

• You should be free of symptoms for at least five days before the challenges of your food start. If your symptoms have improved, start with the discarded foods of your body, "challenging" one meal at a time. Use the Food Diary to keep a record of your symptoms in writing at the end of this paper.

• Add new food to body check every three days. It takes three days to make sure that the symptoms will have time to return if they so wish. You are recommended to eat a small amount on Day 1of re-introduction, have about twice that amount on Day 2, and then an even larger portion on Day 3. See Table 2 for an example calendar. Notice that certain foodstuffs are essential.

It is suitable in small quantities but not in larger quantities. In recognizing these foods, keeping a careful dietary log may be of great help.

• Testing with the purest available form of food is essential. For example, use a pure wheat cereal, which includes wheat only to be tested for wheat. A non-dairy milk alternative such as rice or other milk may be used as long as that milk is not on the "stop" list. Check the milk and cheese in separate occasions. Similar cheeses may or may not have different sensitivities, so it's best to check them separately. Usually, yogurt, cottage cheese, and butter do not have to be tested separately. For chickens, the whites and yolks are separately tested using hard-boiled eggs.

• The food issues should be tackled in the most systematic way possible. Many food elements, such as the proteins casein and whey, and dairy sugar lactose, can be routinely separated by careful challenge planning. Try working with a professional health care provider who can assist you in planning your plan when you suspect a particular component of a food may be a culprit. However, when you exclude an entire food group, it may only be acceptable to challenge the category of one or several different foods, not every single item.

• Delete the item from the diet as soon as the symptom returns, take a note of it, and place it on the "allergic" list in the food diary. If you are unsure of responding to a meal, remove it from your diet and recheck it within 4-5 days. If a food does not cause symptoms during a challenge, it is unlikely to be a problematic food and may eventually be added back to your diet. Nonetheless, don't put the food back during this phase of the program until you've completed the diet and the food challenges. In

283

other words, go back from that diet before it is over to fight for all the foods you have taken out.

Step 4

By eating them, your health care provider can help you plan a way to avoid your symptoms, based on your results. Some things to keep in mind: • This is not a perfect test. It can be extremely difficult to tell for sure that if a particular food is the source. The findings could be interfered with by many other factors (such as a stressful day at work). Try to keep food as consistent as possible when taking the diet.

• Many people have more than one problem with food.

• Make sure you get enough daily care and change your diet over the long run. For example, if you give up dairy, you will need to replace your calcium from other sources such as green leafy vegetables.

• You may need to try multiple different elimination diets before identifying the food problem.

• Many people tolerate this diet well, but if you exercise with the diet many times in an attempt to narrow down the food culprits, the list of allowed foods maybe even smaller. If this happens and you find yourself becoming more intolerant to food or losing enjoyment, please contact a healthcare professional to advise.

• You may have access to certain foods that you are susceptible to on an infrequent or rotational basis. If required, consult with a health care professional to learn how to plan for this.

9.3. Elimination of Inflammation Diet Strategies

Level 1: Simple *(Modified) removal of meat (or dairy and gluten-free)* - This is the lowest-resistance diet. There are two ways to do that. The food, party, or substance in question is focused on the symptoms and alleged culprits. 1. If one item is missing, one food group or one food additive. See Table 1 for the most common culprits in food. This is the easiest diet to adopt, but if symptoms are triggered by more than one food or food group, then this diet may not be helpful. Avoiding only the dairy food category would be perfect for the alleged allergy to lactose. Alternatively, lactase is the enzyme that digests disaccharide lactose and can be administered as an over-the-counter medication. When the lack of lactose causes symptoms to disappear, on occasion, milk can still be enjoyed with the help of lactase.

2. Instead, it removes the two most common culprits in the food group (dairy and wheat). The most common types of food protein that can cause intolerance are the milk protein and wheat gluten in the cow.

• Exclude all dairy products, including milk, butter, sausage, cottage cheese, fruit, cookies, ice cream, and frozen yogurt.

• Exclude gluten, including wheat, spelt, Kamut, oats (allowed to be gluten-free), rye, barley, or malt. This is the principal component of the diet. Substitute products with brown rice, millet, buckwheat, quinoa, gluten-free flour or potato products, tapioca and arrowroot

Level 2: *Low-intensity elimination* - diet In a moderate intensity elimination diet, several foods or classes of foods are removed at once. Ideally, the list of foods excluded is individually modified based on the symptoms and the suspected culprits in the product. For instance, low FODMaP diet may be a good example of symptoms associated with Irritable Bowel Syndrome (IBS) A skilled health care provider can help you identify potential food culprits for your condition or symptoms. Whether complying with the detailed guidelines below and in Table 4 or compiling a custom list. A version of the diet for elimination may be more effective in removing symptoms, as more possible culprits will be removed immediately.

The suggested moderate-intensity elimination diet, in addition to dairy and wheat, excludes meat, all legumes, nuts, several different fruits and vegetables, artificial sweeteners, all animal fats, lots of vegetable fats, chocolate, coffee, tea, soft drinks, and alcohol. This diet will take longer, demanding times to identify the food's culprits. Pay attention to the fact it can be expensive to buy licensed foods.

• Exclude all animal protein; however, where this is not possible or desirable, pork, poultry, and lamb are considered to be a low allergy. Select organic/free-range outlets, wherever possible.

Stop alcohol and caffeine and any papers that may contain these ingredients (including sodas, cold preparations, herbal tinctures).

• Avoid foods containing yeast or foods that promote excessive yeast growth, including processed foods, refined sugars, cheeses, seasonings, peanuts, vinegar, and alcoholic beverages;

• Avoid natural sugars such as chocolate, cookies, and processed foods.

• To drink at least two-quarters of water a day.

Level 3: *The Few-Foods Diet* - This much simpler diet can eat only a small number of foods. This diet should only be followed for a limited period until the food's culprits are detected to ensure no nutritional deficiencies are present.

• This diet is the most restrictive edition and includes only the foods called for in Table 5.

• To help you make the planning process as organized as possible, work with your health care provider;

• This is not a long-term diet consistent with nutrients. In order to ensure proper nutrition, it is necessary to add back foods that do not cause symptoms once the removal time of the diet is over.

9.4. Some Helpful Tips

Looking at food labels, a number of products may be 'disguised.'

If you have an allergy from latex, you can also respond to apple, apricot, avocado, banana, carrot, celery, cherry, chestnut, coconut, fig, shrimp, grape, hazelnut, kiwi, mango, melon, nectarine, papaya, passion fruit, peach, pear, pineapple, plum, potato, rye, shellfish, strawberry, tomato, and wheat.

Conclusion

Inflammation helps the body battle disease and can protect it from injury. In most cases, this is an essential part of the healing process.

However, many people have a medical disorder in which the immune system doesn't function as it should. This failure can lead to permanent or chronically low levels of inflammation. Chronic inflammation occurs in various conditions such as psoriasis, rheumatoid arthritis, and asthma. There's proof that food options can help manage the symptoms. The anti-inflammatory diet favors vegetables and fruit, foods that contain omega-3 fatty acids, whole grains, lean protein, healthy fats, and spices. This prohibits or discourages the use of processed foods, red meats, and alcohol.

The anti-inflammatory diet is a pattern of feeding, rather than a routine. Mediterranean diet and the DASH diet are examples of anti-inflammatory diets.

References

- Anti-inflammatory Diet dishes retrieved from:

https://www.medicalnewstoday.com/articles/322897.php#breakfast

- The elimination diet retrieved from:

https://www.fammed.wisc.edu/files/webfm-uploads/documents/outreach/im/handout_elimination_diet_patient.pdf

- Obesity, inflammation and diet retrieved from:

https://www.ncbi.nlm.nih.gov/pmc/articles/PMC3819692/

- Athlete's guide to fighting elimination retrieved from:

https://www.eleatnutrition.com/blog/inflammation

- The anti-inflammatory lifestyle retrieved from:

https://www.fammed.wisc.edu/files/webfm-uploads/documents/outreach/im/handout_ai_diet_patient.pdf